D1716427

NEW TRENDS IN BRAIN RESEARCH

NEW TRENDS IN BRAIN RESEARCH

F. J. CHEN
EDITOR

Nova Biomedical Books
New York

Copyright © 2006 by Nova Science Publishers, Inc.

For permission to use material from this book please contact us:
Telephone 631-231-7269; Fax 631-231-8175
Web Site: http://www.novapublishers.com

NOTICE TO THE READER

The Publisher has taken reasonable care in the preparation of this book, but makes no expressed or implied warranty of any kind and assumes no responsibility for any errors or omissions. No liability is assumed for incidental or consequential damages in connection with or arising out of information contained in this book. The Publisher shall not be liable for any special, consequential, or exemplary damages resulting, in whole or in part, from the readers' use of, or reliance upon, this material.

This publication is designed to provide accurate and authoritative information with regard to the subject matter covered herein. It is sold with the clear understanding that the Publisher is not engaged in rendering legal or any other professional services. If legal or any other expert assistance is required, the services of a competent person should be sought. FROM A DECLARATION OF PARTICIPANTS JOINTLY ADOPTED BY A COMMITTEE OF THE AMERICAN BAR ASSOCIATION AND A COMMITTEE OF PUBLISHERS.

Library of Congress Cataloging-in-Publication Data
New trends in brain research / F.J. Chen, editor.
p. ; cm.
Includes bibliographical references and index.
ISBN 1-59454-834-X
1. Brain. 2. Brain--Research.   I. Chen, F. J.
[DNLM: 1. Brain--physiopathology. 2. Brain--physiology. WL 300 N5327 2006]
QP376.N495   2006
612.8'2--dc22   2005032211

Published by Nova Science Publishers, Inc. ✤ *New York*

CONTENTS

PREFACE

The brain is omnipresent in bodily functions. Its vast array of responsibilities includes the regulation of all physical movements, memory, learning and emotions, as well as the reception and interpretation of all sensory inputs. These numerous responsibilities require the facility of a very complex organ, and the brain is complex, to the say the least. The brain's complexity provides a constant challenge for scientists to explore new theories. Because of the brain's wide-ranging role in bodily functions these studies have an impact on many other realms of science, such as psychology, neurology, and genetics. This new book features recent studies from this important field of scientific research.

Although the primary concern with respect to hyperbilirubinemia is the potential for neurotoxic effects, general cellular injury also occurs. In chapter 1, the most relevant data obtained by the authors in the field of unconjugated bilirubin (UCB) cytotoxicity is summarized, in an attempt to contribute to a better understanding of the underlying mechanisms of neurotoxicity and cell responsiveness, as well as the role of the most important risk factors for kernicterus. Through studies along the complex alterations in a variety of cell functions, some of the key molecular events and mediators during hyperbilirubinemia are clarified, providing insights into the mechanisms of brain damage by UCB, essential to improve the risk assessment.

In order to go in depth in the understanding of endoreplication, the authors of chapter 2 have revised the available data about endoreplication in invertebrate and vertebrate giant neurons and considered the possible molecular mechanisms responsible for endoreplication. Furthermore, some possible functional significances of neuron endoploidy are also discussed.

Chapter 3 reviews the intracellular signaling mechanism by which neurotrophins prevent ER stress-induced apoptosis in neuronal cells. The authors have recently reported that neurotrophins including NGF (nerve growth factor) and BDNF (brain-derived neurotrophic factor) can suppress ER stress-induced apoptosis in PC12 cells as a model of neurons and in cultured cerebral cortical neurons, respectively. Recently, some genes responsible for neuronal degenerative disorders such as Alzheimer's disease and Parkinson's disease have been identified, and detailed analyses of the molecular mechanisms underlying the onset of neurodegenerative diseases have been carried out. In addition to genetic effectors, environmental effectors acting on cellular homeostatic controls have been analyzed at the molecular level. From these analyses, it has been revealed that endoplasmic reticulum (ER) stress, which is caused by the accumulation of unfolded proteins in the ER, is closely involved in the onset of neurodegenerative processes in neurons. On the other hand, it has also been revealed that neurons die through apoptotic cell death during neurodegenerative processes. However, the molecular mechanism by which ER stress induces apoptosis in neurons remains unclear. In addition, the molecular mechanism behind the processes protecting against ER stress-induced apoptosis in neurons has not been elucidated.

As discussed in chapter 4, sepsis, the systemic response to severe infection, and its complication, the septic shock, show several physiological alterations that include hypotension and changes in hormone secretion. Animal experimental models, such as LPS injection and cecal ligation and puncture can help to understand the pathophysiology of sepsis. Patterns of neurohypophyseal hormone secretion have been reported to be similar in experimental sepsis model and clinical findings. In the early phase of septic shock, elevated vasopressin plasma levels are detected; while in the late phase, these hormone levels are found to be inappropriately low, despite continuing hypotension. In order to understand why these vasopressin levels are so low, recent investigations analyzed neurohypophyseal vasopressin content and corresponding mRNA levels as indices for hormone synthesis. Further studies addressed hormone clearance, sympathetic function, the role of inflammatory mediators and neuronal activation. The neural pathways involved in hypothalamus activation during sepsis have been investigated by using c-*fos* as a marker. These studies revealed the importance of the circumventricular regions and autonomic centers in the medulla oblongata, and point to nitric oxide as the major cause for the deficiency in vasopressin secretion during the late phase of septic shock.

Chapter 5 studies the activation of central α_2-adrenergic/imidazoline receptors which produces several responses that counteract increases in arterial pressure and volume expansion. The α_2-adrenergic/imidazoline agonists like clonidine and moxonidine acting centrally inhibit sympathetic activity, thirst and sodium appetite and induce diuresis and natriuresis. The involvement of central α_2-adrenergic vs. imidazoline receptors has been subjected to controversies, but there is also evidence that both receptors may interact in some of these responses. A stronger inhibitory effect on thirst and sodium appetite is produced by mixed α_2-adrenergic/imidazoline agonists, than by selective α_2-adrenergic agonists; an effect likely independent from activation of presynaptic α_2-adrenergic receptors. Mixed α_2-adrenergic/imidazoline antagonists are also much more potent than non-imidazoline antagonists to inhibit the agonists. Although the anti-hypertensive effects of α_2-adrenergic/imidazoline agonists is dependent on hindbrain areas, injections of the α_2-adrenergic/imidazoline agonists inhibit water intake and induces diuresis and natriuresis when injected into the lateral ventricle (LV), but not into the 4th ventricle (4th V). On the other hand inhibition of sodium appetite is produced by injections of α_2-adrenergic/imidazoline agonists into the LV or 4th V. In spite of the established inhibitory effect of centrally acting α_2-adrenergic/imidazoline agonists on water and NaCl intake, recent results from our laboratory have shown that injections of moxonidine or clonidine into the lateral parabrachial nucleus (LPBN) strongly increase hypertonic NaCl intake and abolish the effects of the activation of the inhibitory LPBN serotonergic mechanisms. Therefore, the central activation of α_2-adrenergic/imidazoline receptors through the ventricular system inhibits sodium intake, but activation of the same type of receptors in the LPBN strongly increases sodium intake probably by the blockade of the serotonergic inhibitory mechanisms.

The aim of the work presented in chapter 6 was to investigate locomotor responses in Wistar rats in normal and reverse light-dark cycles, as well as the effect of different doses of alcohol. Low doses of alcohol have been reported to induce psychomotor activation in rodents, whereas high doses produce sedation. However, locomotor responses to alcohol may be influenced by different factors, including the dose and route of administration, the duration of drug exposure, the distinct sensitivity of rodent strains, the light-dark cycle and stressful situations. Behavioral responses were assessed in an activity meter and scores of slow and fast horizontal movements, as well as slow and fast stereotyped movements were recorded. The results suggest that stimulant alcohol effects may be mainly due to fast horizontal and fast stereotyped movements. In contrast, the sedative alcohol effects may involve similar contributions of slow and fast horizontal, as well as fast stereotyped movements. Alcohol behavioral effects may be closely related to activation of brain dopaminergic circuits.

The authors of chapter 7 have used immunocytochemistry to analyze expression of BCL-2, MCL-1, BCL-X_S, BAX and BAD of the BCL-2 family of proteins and of caspase-1, -2_L, -3, 6, -8 and -9 of the caspase family in frontal cortex slices of eight postmortem brains of sporadic CJD patients and three neuropathologically unaltered controls. Neuronal apoptosis in Creutzfeldt-Jakob disease (CJD) is well documented. However, little is known about associated signaling pathways. Recent results have demonstrated close interactions of cyclooxygenases, BCL-2 family members and caspases in the regulation of survival of central nervous system cells including neurons and their involvement in the modulation of apoptosis in diseases of the brain. Their localization in brains of CJD patients, however, remains unresolved. Double labeling experiments confirmed the neuronal origin of BCL-2 and caspase family expressing cells. They observed accumulation of antiapoptotic MCL-1 (P= 0.004), proapoptotic BCL-X_S (P=0.016) and BAX (P=0.016) and of caspase-6 (P<0.001) and –8 (P<0.001) in cortical neurons of CJD compared to controls. Immunoreactivity of the other analyzed BCL-2 and caspase family members was only rarely observed in singular neurons in both, CJD patients and controls. Abundant data has previously demonstrated that effectors of cyclooxygenases, nonsteroidal anti-inflammatory drugs, induce the alteration of BCL-2 and caspase family members to influence cellular survival. Cyclooxygenases (COX) mediate inflammation, immunomodulation, blood flow, apoptosis and fever in various diseases of the brain. While COX-2 is cytokine-inducible, COX-1 is expressed by macrophages/microglial cells that accumulate in pathological foci. In a previous report, the authors observed significant accumulation of COX-1 in macrophages/microglial cells adjacent to neurons in brains of patients with Creutzfeldt-Jakob disease. COX-2 was predominantly observed in neurons, and their number was significantly higher compared to controls. Although formal proof is lacking, the data may indicate that NSAIDs may influence the course of CJD. However, the cyclooxygenase-BCL-2 family-caspase pathway is a modulator not only of apoptosis, but also of cellular differentiation, immune-reaction and angiogenesis. Additional data needs to be acquired to justify clinical trials using NSAIDs in these patients.

The study presented in chapter 8 is on the topic of gliomas which are the most common type of primary malignant brain tumors in Malaysia. Several ideas have emerged about the genetic alterations occurring in human cancers and how they contribute to tumorigenesis. The role of common genetic alterations in determining the range of individual susceptibility within the population are being increasingly recognized. The accumulation of genetic alterations are thought to drive the progression of normal cells through hyperplastic and dysplastic stages to invasive cancer and, finally, metastatic disease. With regards to that, abundant research has been aggressively carried out, focusing on the potential roles of genes which are important in cell cycle progression as well as apoptotic pathways. The results have revealed *PTEN* and *p53* genes mutations to be found in mostly high grade gliomas. Loss of heterozygosity (LOH) and telomerase activities were also found in high grade glioma cases, suggesting that those actions might contribute to brain tumorigenesis in Malaysia especially amongst the Malay population. The identification of genes and pathways involved would enhance our understanding of the biology of this process. It would also provide new targets for early diagnosis and facilitate treatment design for example in developing DNA vaccine as an anti-cancer agent and virus therapy which has shown promise as a cancer treatment in Malaysia.

Chapter 9 presents a methodology for functional brain mapping through the integration of optical topographic maps (OTM) with anatomical magnetic resonance imaging (MRI). The topographic images are mapped to both the skull and cortical surface of the brain. Eight subjects underwent an MRI and optical topography system (OTS) exams, during which anatomical MR images and optical topographic maps were acquired. In order to map the motor functional areas in the brain, a functional experiment is performed by using the ETG-100 OTS and is based on a repeated finger-tapping task alternated with relaxed states. The integration process involves estimating the probes location on the MRI head model and warping the 2D topographic images on the 3D MRI head/brain model. After integrating OTS with MRI a movie depicting the changes of the brain activation is played on the MRI head model. A graphical user interface (GUI) is developed to integrate the above modalities and serve as an application platform for neuroscience studies and for assisting neurosurgeons at localizing key functional regions in the brain.

In: New Trends in Brain Research
Editor: F. J. Chen, pp. 1-38

ISBN 1-59454-834-X
© 2006 Nova Science Publishers, Inc.

Chapter I

CELL RESPONSE TO HYPERBILIRUBINEMIA: A JOURNEY ALONG KEY MOLECULAR EVENTS

Maria Alexandra Brito, Rui F. M. Silva and Dora Brites

Centro de Patogénese Molecular (UBMBE), Faculdade de Farmácia, University of Lisbon, Lisbon, Portugal

ABSTRACT

Jaundice occurs in approximately 60% of healthy term neonates without sequelae. However, in some infants hyperbilirubinemia can cause encephalopathy or kernicterus, especially in the presence of aggravating conditions such as prematurity, infection, acidosis and diminished albumin binding capacity and/or affinity. Evidence of minor neurologic dysfunction in moderately jaundiced infants and recent resurgence of kernicterus has brought the clinical management of hyperbilirubinemia to daylight again. Although the primary concern with respect to hyperbilirubinemia is the potential for neurotoxic effects, general cellular injury also occurs. In this book chapter, it will be summarized the most relevant data obtained by our group in the field of unconjugated bilirubin (UCB) cytotoxicity, in an attempt to contribute to a better understanding of the underlying mechanisms of neurotoxicity and cell responsiveness, as well as the role of the most important risk factors for kernicterus.

Our initial studies, performed using the red blood cell as a model of cellular binding and toxicity, showed that *in vitro* exposure to UCB induces crenation and profound disturbances of cell integrity. These perturbations increase with the UCB to albumin molar ratio and with acidosis, pointing to diacid UCB as the cytotoxic species and implicating the UCB precipitates in the irreversible mechanisms of cytotoxicity. This late finding was corroborated by the inability of albumin to remove UCB from erythrocyte membranes. In line with the *in vitro* studies, blood samples from moderately jaundiced neonates present similar morphological and structural alterations. Interestingly, they also reveal higher levels of membrane-bound hemoglobin, an indicator of oxidative stress. In agreement with this observation, and despite the protective role of nanomolar concentrations of UCB, high levels of this pigment induce oxidative stress in several other experimental systems, namely synaptosomal vesicles, isolated brain mitochondria and whole nerve cells, where production of reactive oxygen species, oxidation of proteins and lipids, and disruption of glutathione metabolism were observed. The disorder of the redox status is accompanied by an impairment of membrane dynamic properties, such as phospholipid packing, protein motion, and polarity of the membrane microenvironment. Oxidative injury to synaptosomes is further linked to a reduced activity of membrane ATPases, which shall be implicated in the UCB-induced disruption of calcium homeostasis. Oxidative stress and intracellular calcium accumulation are usually associated with an inflammatory response, extracellular accumulation of glutamate, or even cell death, events also induced by UCB in nerve cells. In fact, exposure of astrocytes to UCB promotes the secretion of TNF-α and IL-1β, increases the extracellular concentration of glutamate, therefore engendering excitotoxicity, and induces nerve cell death by both necrosis and apoptosis. Despite the UCB ability to damage both neurons and astrocytes, the different response of these cellular types point to distinct pathways of neurotoxicity, where oxidative injury emerges as a key factor. In fact, our newest data showed that UCB promotes protein oxidation and lipid peroxidation in neurons, but not in astrocytes. Moreover, astrocytes are resistant to oxidative injury even in the presence of endotoxin, which was shown to have additive effects on the secretion of pro-inflammatory cytokines and cell death. Finally, fetal cells by binding UCB more avidly and showing early signs of decreased viability appear as sensitive targets for UCB toxicity, while the enhanced inflammatory response by immature nerve cells, provide a basis for prematurity as a risk factor for kernicterus.

In conclusion, through this journey along the complex alterations in a variety of cell functions, some of the key molecular events and mediators during hyperbilirubinemia are clarified, providing insights into the mechanisms of brain damage by UCB, essential to improve the risk assessment.

BILIRUBIN: GENERAL PRINCIPLES

Bilirubin is the principal end product of the degradation of heme moiety of hemoglobin and other hemoproteins in mammals. It is formed in the reticuloendothelial system as a result of a multistep process in which two enzymatic systems are involved: the microsomal heme oxygenase, followed by the ubiquitous cytosolic biliverdin reductase (Figure 1). In this process, the porphyrin ring of heme is first opened by enzymatic oxidation, leading to the formation of a green linear tetrapyrrolic pigment, designated biliverdin, and to the release of equimolar amounts of CO and iron which are excreted by lungs and reutilized, respectively. Biliverdin is then rapidly and quantitatively reduced to bilirubin, a yellow-orange pigment (Berk and Noyer, 1994).

Due to its structure (Figure 2), in which internal hydrogen bonding masks the propionic acid side chains, bilirubin is poorly soluble in aqueous medium (<70 nM) (Berk and Noyer, 1994; Ostrow et al., 1994). Therefore, over 99.9% bilirubin is transported in the blood tightly bound to albumin (Figure 3), a carrier molecule with a single high affinity binding site for one bilirubin molecule, and biotransformation is required for excretion from the body (Berk and Noyer, 1994; Gourley, 1997; Ostrow et al., 2004). After uptake by the hepatocyte, which occurs at least in part via carrier mediated mechanisms, the pigment is transported by a protein carrier, known as glutathione S-transferase, ligandin or Y protein. Once within the endoplasmic reticulum, bilirubin is conjugated with either one or two molecules of glucuronic acid, by the action of the enzyme bilirubin UDP-glucuronosyl transferase. These mono- and di-glucuronides display high polarity, which renders them water soluble and unable to diffuse across membranes, and allows their secretion into bile via the canalicular multispecific organic anion transporter, MRP2/Mrp2.

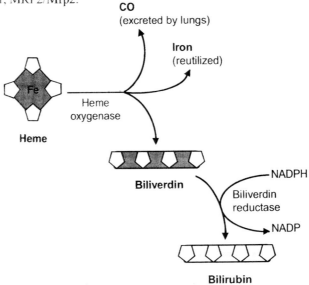

Figure 1. Schematic representation of bilirubin synthesis from heme catabolism. Heme ring is opened by heme oxygenase yelding biliverdin and releasing equimolar amounts of carbon monoxide (CO) and iron. The green pigment biliverdin is reduced to the yellow-orange pigment bilirubin by biliverdin reductase.

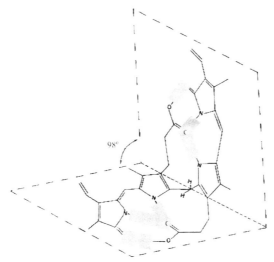

Figure 2. Structure of unconjugated bilirubin. The molecule consists of two rigid, planar dipyrrole units joined by a methylene (-CH$_2$) bridge at carbon 10, and is stabilized by hydrogen bonds (highlighted). Adapted from Ostrow *et al.* (1994).

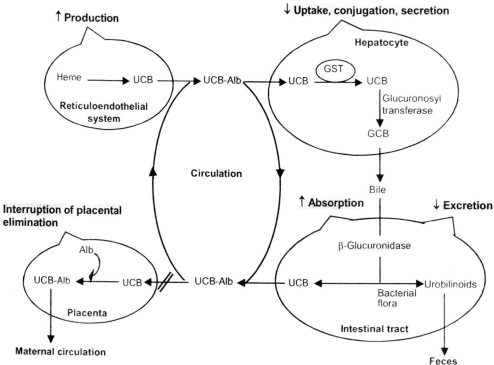

Figure 3. Schematic representation of bilirubin metabolism, highlighting the particular features of fetal and neonatal life. UCB, unconjugated bilirubin; Alb, albumin; GST, glutathione S-transferase; GCB, glucuronide-conjugated bilirubin.

Conjugated bilirubin excreted in bile passes through the small intestine without significant absorption. In the colon, it is both deconjugated, presumably by the bacterial β-glucuronidase, and degraded by other bacterial enzymes to a large family of reduction-oxidation products, collectively known as urobilinoids, which are mostly excreted by feces (Figure 3).

PATHOPHYSIOLOGY OF NEONATAL JAUNDICE

In fetal life, bilirubin production begins as early as 12 weeks' gestation (Reiser, 2004). Despite the limited excretory function of the fetal liver, the presence of β-glucuronidase and the absence of bacterial flora in the fetal bowel enable bilirubin to remain as unconjugated bilirubin (UCB), therefore allowing its passage to maternal circulation (Figure 3). At birth, this placental protection is suddenly lost, just when an acute increase in production of UCB occurs, due to the shorter red blood cell (RBC) life span of newborns (70-90 vs. 120 days in adults), especially if prematures. In addition, the newborn has to use its own immature mechanisms for hepatic uptake, conjugation and biliary secretion of bilirubin, reason why a significant retention of UCB occurs, even in healthy term neonates (Blanckaert and Fevery, 1990; Gourley, 1997; Reiser, 2004). Such retention is further enhanced by the absence of anaerobic ileo-colonic flora in the newborn infant, leading to more unmetabolized UCB available for intestinal absorption, thus increasing the entero-hepatic circulation of UCB

(Vítek *et al.*, 2000). As a result, virtually all newborn infants will have mild to moderate elevated serum UCB levels (less than 170 μM) within the first days of life, a condition known as "physiologic jaundice". Therefore, this neonatal jaundice reflects the transition from intrauterine to extrauterine bilirubin metabolism and is linked to normal development; it is considered benign, and is usually resolved by the end of the first week of life with no treatment requirement (Ostrow *et al.*, 2003; Reiser, 2004).

Hyperbilirubinemia: The Two Faces of a Coin

UCB has long been regarded as a waste product, lacking any clear physiologic role. However, accumulating evidence strongly suggests that UCB is a potent antioxidant, even when bound to albumin (Clark *et al.*, 2000; Doré *et al.*, 1999; McDonagh, 1990; Stocker *et al.*, 1987). In fact, several studies have shown that UCB provides primary protection from injury resulting from oxidation, such as ischemia-related injuries (Doré *et al.*, 2000), as well as the risk of coronary artery disease (Mayer, 2000) and cancer (Keshavan *et al.*, 2004; Zucker *et al.*, 2004). The ability of low nanomolar concentrations of UCB to overcome large amounts of oxidants was explained by a redox cycling mechanism, whereas biliverdin reductase plays a key role (Barañano *et al.*, 2002). Through this catalytic cycle, UCB is oxidized at the central carbon (C-10) to biliverdin by oxidant species, neutralizing their toxicity, and then is regenerated by the action of biliverdin reductase (Figure 4). As this cycle is repeated, the antioxidant effect of UCB is multiplied, rendering UCB as a major physiologic antioxidant cytoprotectant (Barañano *et al.*, 2002).

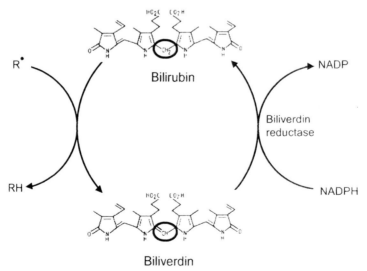

Figure 4. Amplification of the antioxidant properties of unconjugated bilirubin by a redox cycling. Large amounts of oxidant species (R•) can be neutralized (RH) through bilirubin oxidation to biliverdin, which is rapidly reduced back to bilirubin by biliverdin reductase.

Because of the antioxidant properties of low UCB concentrations, it is nowadays believed that physiologic jaundice may have inherent benefits. However, in some newborn infants, plasma UCB levels can increase dramatically owing to impaired postnatal maturation of hepatic transport or conjugation of UCB, and/or enhanced entero-hepatic circulation of UCB, or augmented hemolysis. If untreated, hyperbilirubinemia can cause toxicity to the basal ganglia and various brainstem nuclei, leading to acute UCB encephalopathy or kernicterus, depending on whether the clinical manifestations of neurological damage are reversible or progress to chronic and permanent clinical sequelae, or even death (American Academy of Pediatrics, 2004).

Resurgence of Kernicterus

The recent reports of kernicterus (Ebbesen, 2000; Hansen, 2000; Maisels and Newman, 1998; Maisels and Newman, 1995; Mollen et al., 2004; Palmer et al., 2004), after a 20 years period where this pathological condition had nearly disappeared in full-term infants (Blanckaert and Fevery, 1990; Dennery et al., 2001; Gourley, 1997; Kaplan and Hammerman, 2004; Reiser, 2004), brought the pathological conditions associated with hyperbilirubinemia to daylight again, and reawakened the interest in the understanding of the mechanisms underlying UCB neurotoxicity. To the reemergence of kernicterus shall have accounted the early hospital discharge of term infants and the increased survival of prematurely born infants (Dennery et al., 2001; Gourley, 1997; Maisels and Newman, 1998), together with the implementation of kinder and gentler approaches to the management of neonatal jaundice (Newman and Maisels, 1992). The evidence of minor neurologic dysfunctions throughout the first year of life in children that have presented a moderate neonatal hyperbilirubinemia, indicated that the serum UCB level is not the only hazardous factor to consider in the management of neonatal hyperbilirubinemia. Therefore, there is now a growing concern to elucidate the role of other risk factors, such as the albumin binding capacity and/or affinity, acidosis, sepsis, and prematurity (American Academy of Pediatrics, 2004), in order to identify the newborn infants at risk of neurological damage by UCB.

Impairment of Cell Function by Unconjugated Bilirubin

Although the primary concern with respect to hyperbilirubinemia is the potential for neurotoxic effects, general cellular injury also occurs, as pointed out by the panoply of toxic events occurring in different study models. The first experimental studies of UCB toxicity pointed to an inhibition of respiration in brain homogenates and uncoupling of oxidative phosphorylation (Day, 1954; Ernster and Zetterström, 1956). Results from several other studies indicate that UCB is toxic to various cellular functions, as evidenced by the impairment of DNA and protein synthesis (Day, 1954; Schiff et al., 1985; Yamada et al., 1977), interference with neurotransmitter metabolism (Day, 1954; Ochoa et al., 1993; Roseth et al., 1998), and depression of the immune response (Haga et al., 1996; Vetvicka et al., 1991). The alterations in membrane potential, transport and enzymatic systems (Karp, 1979; Mayor et al., 1986; Tsakiris, 1993) point to the disruption of the cell membrane structure as a common denominator underlying the mechanisms of cytotoxicity by UCB. It was even pointed out that the amount of UCB bound to the membrane, rather than its concentration in the medium, determines the magnitude of the toxic effect (Brodersen, 1981).

THE HUMAN RBC AS A MODEL OF UNCONJUGATED BILIRUBIN BINDING AND TOXICITY

Our initial studies of UCB cellular binding and toxicity were performed using the human RBC as a model, due to its accessibility, the absence of intracellular organelles, and the similarities of some membrane components with those of other cell types (Bennett, 1985). Moreover, UCB binding to RBC has been considered a sensitive indicator of cellular affinity and toxicity (Barthez et al., 1982; Bouillerot et al., 1981; Malik et al., 1986), and proposed as a criterion to assess the risk of bilirubin encephalopathy (Kaufmann et al., 1967; Malik et al., 1986).

Unconjugated Bilirubin Toxicity Involves Profound Disturbances of Cell Integrity

As shown in Figure 5, exposure of human RBC to high concentrations of free UCB (171 µM) leads to the appearance of echinocytic forms, which may derive from an evagination of the membrane as a result of the interaction of UCB with the outer leaflet of the bilayer. The shape changes, expressed quantitatively as the morphological index, are accompanied by the release of membrane phospholipids and most likely result in a subsequent and irreversible stage of UCB toxicity that culminates in cell lysis and appearance of hemoglobin-depleted cell-like vesicles. In fact, crenation is more evident in the 5-30 min after UCB addition, where hemolysis is virtually absent, but the extent of shape changes becomes less pronounced as hemolysis starts to occur (Brites et al., 1997). Therefore, echinocytosis and membrane deposition of UCB, leading to loss of both phospholipids and hemoglobin, as well as cell destruction, are different stages of UCB interaction with the RBC membrane (Brito et al., 1996). Interestingly, the early stage of UCB toxicity, corresponding to cell crenation, is preferentially shown by younger cells, while the final and irreversible step, probably due to UCB acid aggregation, is facilitated by an increased age of RBC (Brites et al., 1997).

UCB also perturbs the normal distribution of membrane phospholipids. In fact, we have observed that the pigment not only induces marked alterations in the membrane content of several classes of phospholipids, but also leads to the translocation of the inner leaflet aminophospholipids to the outer leaflet of the membrane (Brito et al., 2002). These alterations point to an accelerated ageing of RBC exposed to UCB, which was referred to be accompanied by loss of components as a result of membrane fragmentation and release of vesicles (Greenwalt and Dumaswala, 1988). The RBC that became senescent by UCB interaction shall be recognized and removed from circulation. This assumption is convincingly documented by the externalization of phosphatidylserine induced by UCB (Brito et al., 2002), which seems to constitute a signal for the phagocyte engulfment by macrophages.

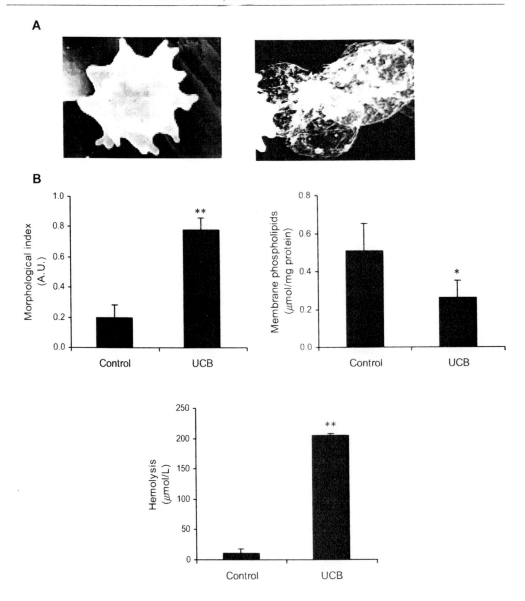

Figure 5. Unconjugated bilirubin induces morphological alterations, disruption of membrane structure and hemolysis of human erythrocytes. Erythrocytes were incubated in the absence (0 μM; control) or in the presence of 171 μM purified unconjugated bilirubin (UCB), at pH 7.4, for 3 h, at 37°C. Morphological analysis, performed by scanning electron microscopy, revealed the presence of echinocytes and hemoglobin-depleted cell-like vesicles in UCB-treated erythrocytes (A). The extent of shape changes was quantitatively expressed as the morphological index, and membrane phospholipids and hemolysis were determined as lipid phosphorus and hemoglobin release, respectively (B). *P<0.05 and **P<0.01 from control. Derived from data of Brito *et al.* (1996) and from Brites *et al.* (1997).

Increased Levels of Serum Bilirubin and Acidosis Aggravate the Extent of Cell Damage

The extent of the previously mentioned effects on human erythrocytes, namely the shape changes and hemolysis, as well as the release of phospholipids and their redistribution, increase with the UCB to human serum albumin (HSA) molar ratio (Figure 6), as would be anticipated. In fact, in blood plasma UCB circulates almost entirely bound to HSA, so that, with a normal albumin concentration of 435 μM (3 g/100 mL) as much as 435 μM (25 mg/100 mL) of UCB will be transported. However, as the UCB to HSA molar ratio exceeds the unity, the albumin capacicity for UCB binding is surpassed and the amount of unbound UCB sharply rises (Brodersen, 1981). In these conditions, the free fraction of UCB, which is mainly in the non ionised (protonated diacid) form at physiological pH, can passively diffuse across membranes and impair cell viability (Ostrow et al., 2004). Our findings assume a particular relevance since a decreased albumin concentration and a lower affinity and/or

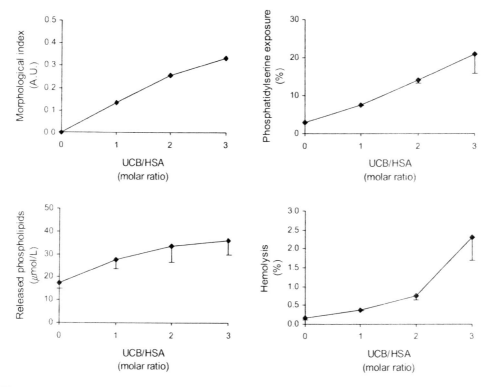

Figure 6. Dose-response of human erythrocytes to unconjugated bilirubin-induced morphological alterations, disruption of membrane structure and hemolysis. Erythrocytes were incubated in the absence (control) or in the presence of 114-340 μM purified unconjugated bilirubin (UCB), at different UCB to human serum albumin (HAS) molar ratio values, at pH 7.4, for 4 h, at 37°C. Morphological analysis was performed by scanning electron microscopy and the extent of shape changes was quantitatively expressed as the morphological index; membrane phospholipids, phosphatidylserine exposure, and hemolysis were determined as lipid phosphorus, annexin V binding and hemoglobin release, respectively. Statistically significant differences from control were observed for all the UCB/HSA molar ratios. Derived from data of Brito et al. (2000).

capacity for UCB binding is frequently found in neonates, especially in the low weight premature infants (Cashore, 1980; Kaplan and Hammerman, 2004). Furthermore, the already statistically significant effects observed at an UCB to HSA molar ratio of one (Figure 6) provide an explanation for the manifestations of toxicity, and even cases of kernicterus, occurring in severely jaundiced newborns (Gourley, 1997; Kaplan and Hammerman, 2004; Watchko and Maisels, 2003), where this ratio value can be attained.

Another frequent condition during neonatal life usually associated with an aggravation of UCB cytotoxicity is acidosis (Brodersen, 1981). To this fact shall contribute the protonation of the propionic acid residues of the UCB molecule in an acidic medium, and the aggregation of the so-called acid UCB within the membrane, in contrast with the ionisation of the side chain(s) at alkaline pH values that render the molecule more soluble and less toxic (Ostrow *et al.*, 1994). In our studies (Figure 7), acidosis revealed to enhance the extent of morphological alterations and hemolysis, probably as a reflex of an increased binding of UCB to

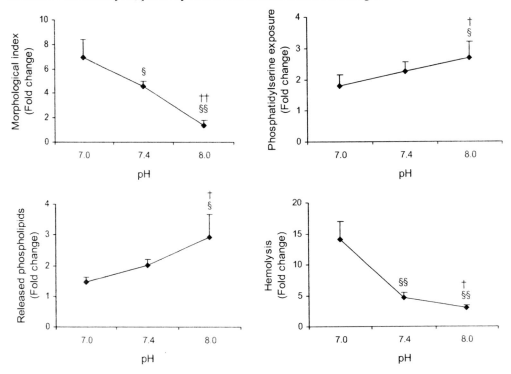

Figure 7. Unconjugated bilirubin-induced morphological alterations, disruption of membrane structure and hemolysis are differently affected by acidosis. Human erythrocytes were incubated in the absence (control) or in the presence of 340 µM purified unconjugated bilirubin (UCB), at a UCB to human serum albumin molar ratio of 3, for 4 h, at 37°C, at different pH values. Morphological analysis was performed by scanning electron microscopy and the extent of shape changes was quantitatively expressed as the morphological index; membrane phospholipids, phosphatidylserine exposure, and hemolysis were determined as lipid phosphorus, annexin V binding and hemoglobin release, respectively. Statistically significant differences vs. respective control were obtained for all the parameters except for morphological index at pH 8.0 and phosphatidylserine exposure at pH 7.0; fold changes were calculated based on corresponding controls. §P<0.05 and §§P<0.01 from pH 7.0; †P<0.05 and ††P<0.01 from pH 7.4. Derived from data of Brito and Brites (2003).

which is in agreement with previous reports (Bratlid, 1972; Rashid *et al.*, 2000). On the other hand, an acidic medium lessens the loss of phospholipids, as well as their redistribution, probably by promoting the formation of UCB complexes with membrane phospholipids. The aggregation of UCB dimers at the membrane level, progressively originating acid UCB microcrystals (Vázquez *et al.*, 1988), shall be responsible for the irreversible damage that culminates in cell lysis. Therefore, these data provide a basis for the role of acidosis as an aggravating condition of hyperbilirubinemia, pointing to acid UCB as the cytotoxic species, and rendering UCB precipitates as the entities mainly responsible for the demolition of the membrane architecture (Brito and Brites, 2003)

Erythrocyte-bound Unconjugated Bilirubin is only Partially Recovered by Albumin

In the clinical management of jaundice, a crucial aspect is the reversibility of the toxic manifestations of UCB by therapeutics, such as albumin administration. Nevertheless, the wash of erythrocytes with albumin after incubation with UCB, although decreasing the extent of shape changes, is not able to completely restore the normal morphology (Figure 8A).

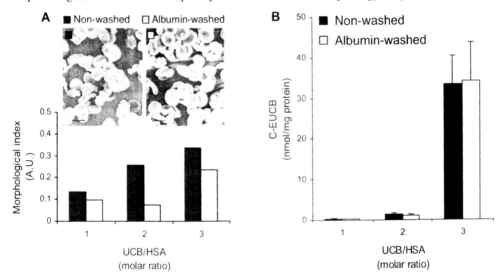

Figure 8. Albumin is unable to completely reverse the morphological alterations induced by unconjugated bilirubin and to extract all the erythrocyte-bound unconjugated bilirubin, which is only recovered by chloroform extraction. Human erythrocytes were incubated in the absence (control) or in the presence of 114-340 μM purified unconjugated bilirubin (UCB) and 114 μM human serum albumin (HSA), corresponding to different UCB/HSA molar ratio values, at pH 7.4, for 4 h, at 37°C. Morphological analysis was performed by scanning electron microscopy and the extent of shape changes was quantitatively expressed as the morphological index (A); chloroform extractable erythrocyte-bound UCB (C-EUCB) was determined in non-washed and albumin-washed erythrocytes using chloroform as a solvent for UCB (B). C-EUCB was not detected in control assays and no statistically significant differences were obtained between the C-EUCB levels of non-washed and albumin-washed erythrocytes. Bar: 10 μm. Derived from data of Brito et al. (2000).

These observations indicate that only the superficial and non-aggregated UCB molecules are taken off by albumin, and that no other than the initial stages of membrane toxicity can be entirely reverted by albumin. By contrast, the UCB aggregates involved in the irreversible mechanisms of UCB-induced toxicity can only be recovered by solubilization with chloroform (Figure 8B). These findings indicate that the determination of chloroform-extractable erythrocyte bound-UCB (C-EUCB) is a more reliable technique to evaluate the extent of UCB binding to erythrocyte membranes than the albumin-extractable erythrocyte bound-UCB (A-EUCB) (Moreau-Clevede and Pays, 1979), so far used. Therefore, appreciation of C-EUCB levels may add valuable information to improve the assessment of the risk of UCB cytotoxicity (Brito *et al.*, 2000).

UNCONJUGATED BILIRUBIN BINDING TO HUMAN ERYTHROCYTES DURING NEONATAL JAUNDICE ELICITS TOXICITY

In line with the *in vitro* studies, the examination of blood samples obtained from moderately jaundiced neonates (185 µM UCB; UCB to albumin molar ratio of 0.4), revealed the presence of echinocytosis, together with a decreased content of membrane phospholipids (Brito *et al.*, 1996). As expected, the magnitude of the effects observed in the physiologic and reversible neonatal hyperbilirubinemia (Figure 9) is lower than that found in the *in vitro* study (Figure 5), which intends to mimic the irreversible pathological condition of kernicterus. To this fact accounts the absence of albumin in the later study, which leads to much higher levels of free UCB and favors its interaction with the membranes, despite the same range of concentrations of the pigment (<200 µM).

Interestingly, jaundiced neonates exhibit significantly higher levels of membrane-bound hemoglobin, as compared with healthy babies or adults (Figure 9). This finding reinforces the already mentioned accelerated ageing of erythrocytes exposed to UCB (Brito *et al.*, 2002), since hemoglobin binding to membranes was shown to increase during *in vivo* erythrocyte senescence (Rettig *et al.*, 1999). Furthermore, this observation raises the hypothesis that high levels of UCB may induce oxidative injury, considering that membrane-bound hemoglobin increases with the level of oxidative stress (Sharma and Premachandra, 1991).

Unconjugated Bilirubin-induced Toxicity is Exacerbated in Human Neonatal Erythrocytes

UCB binding and its pernicious effects are exacerbated in neonatal RBC (Brito, 2001). In effect, cells obtained from the umbilical cord blood suffered more drastic changes than those form adults, following exposure to the pigment (UCB to HSA molar ratio of 3), as shown by the higher distortion of morphology and depletion of membrane phospholipids, together with the more marked disruption of the normal bilayer asymmetry indicated by the increased externalization of phosphatidylserine (Figure 10). The proneness of neonatal cells to suffer such profound disturbances of membrane structure shall lead to a further acceleration of the UCB-induced erythrocyte senescence. As a result, the hemolysis is nearly 5-times greater than that of adults. Underlying the vulnerability of neonatal cells to the injurious effects of UCB shall be a different binding and accommodation of the pigment within the membrane, as indicated by the opposite profiles of A-EUCB and C-EUCB in neonates vs. adults. Actually, erythrocytes from adults bind mainly UCB monomers at a superficial level of the membrane and, thus, UCB is easily removed by albumin washing. Cells from the umbilical cord blood, although presenting less A-EUCB, contain a bigger fraction of the pigment inaccessible to albumin, probably as aggregates of acid UCB with the membrane phospholipids, which is only recovered by chloroform. This C-EUCB presumably corresponds to the fraction implicated in the enhanced irreversible toxicity in neonatal cells. Our observations are in line with the higher capacity for UCB incorporation referred by Vázquez *et al.* (1988) in synaptosomal plasma membrane vesicles of neonatal rats.

Collectively, these data indicate that erythrocytes from newborn infants, by binding UCB more avidly and showing signs of a marked viability decline, represent sensitive targets of UCB toxicity, thus playing a pivotal role during hyperbilirubinemia. The enhanced senescence rate shall favor erythrophagocytosis, therefore contributing to raise hemolysis that further aggravates neonatal jaundice through a vicious circle.

UNCONJUGATED BILIRUBIN IMPAIRS MEMBRANE DYNAMIC PROPERTIES IN SEVERAL EXPERIMENTAL MODELS

Human Erythrocyte Right-side-out Vesicles

Previous data have pointed to the cell membrane as a primary target of UCB cytotoxicity. To clarify whether UCB has a special avidity for different regions of the membrane, namely the lipid-water interface, the carbonyl or the methylene chain regions or, eventually, the middle of the bilayer, we performed electron paramagnetic resonance (EPR) spectroscopy analysis of right-side-out vesicles, using several spin labeled phospholipids, in order to selectively establish the perturbations of UCB on membrane dynamic properties at different depths of the leaflet (Brito *et al.*, 2001).

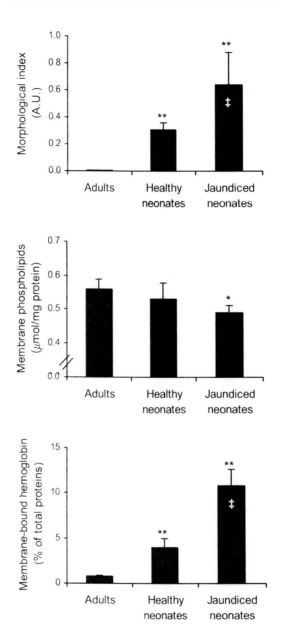

Figure 9. Human erythrocytes from jaundiced neonates present alterations of morphology and membrane lipid composition, and bind hemoglobin avidly. Human erythrocytes were obtained from moderately jaundiced neonates (185 μM unconjugated bilirubin; bilirubin/albumin molar ratio of 0.4), as well as from the umbilical cord blood of healthy newborn infants, and adult donors. Morphological analysis was performed by scanning electron microscopy and the extent of shape changes was quantitatively expressed as the morphological index; membrane phospholipids were determined as lipid phosphorus, and membrane-bound hemoglobin was evaluated based on the peroxidase activity of hemoproteins. *P<0.05 and **P<0.01 from adults; ‡P<0.01 from healthy neonates. Derived from data of Brito *et al.* (1996) and Brito (2001).

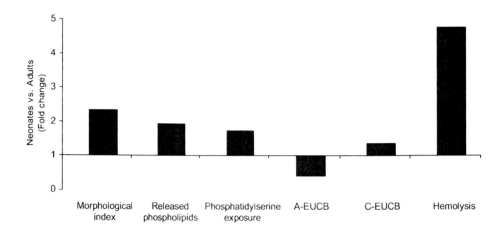

Figure 10. Unconjugated bilirubin-induced toxicity is exacerbated in human neonatal erythrocytes as compared to adults. Human erythrocytes were obtained from either adult donors or umbilical cord blood of healthy neonates and incubated in the absence (control) or presence of 340 μM purified unconjugated bilirubin (UCB), at a UCB to human serum albumin molar ratio of 3, at pH 7.4, for 4 h, at 37°C. Morphological analysis was performed by scanning electron microscopy and the extent of shape changes was quantitatively expressed as the morphological index; membrane phospholipids, phosphatidylserine exposure, and hemolysis were determined as lipid phosphorus, annexin V binding and hemoglobin release, respectively. Erythrocyte-bound UCB was determined by albumin extraction (A-EUCB), and the amount of the pigment not removed by albumin was recovered using chloroform as a solvent (C-EUCB). Statistically significant differences were obtained for all the parameters vs. respective control, in both groups, and between adults and neonates. Derived from data of Brito (2001).

Interestingly, UCB leads to a dual effect in the membrane lipid package and polarity, decreasing the phospholipids mobility and the polarity environment at carbon number 5 region, while inducing their increase at C-7, and less markedly at C-12 and C-16 (Figure 11). These results indicate that accommodation of UCB occurs at C-5, therefore decreasing the already low chain motion of phospholipids. The intercalation of foreign molecules shall render the inner regions of the leaflet more fluid and more permeable to water diffusion, as a second-hand effect. The decrease in the extent of membrane perturbation from C-7 to C-16 may be understood as a wave progressively attenuating as the distance from the primary interaction target increases. Thus, from our data we may conclude that at least a portion of the UCB molecule interacts to some extent with the hydrocarbon core at the superficial regions of the membrane, in agreement with previous studies (Cestaro *et al.*, 1983; Zakim and Wong, 1990; Zucker *et al.*, 1992), and sustaining the appearance of echinocytic forms following exposure to UCB. Moreover, the solubility characteristics of the molecule would not favor its intercalation between the phospholipid acyl chains (Brodersen, 1979), while the lack of effect at C-16 is also consistent with the accommodation of UCB in lipid bilayers at regions different from the methyl terminal end of the acyl chain (Cestaro *et al.*, 1983; Zakim and Wong, 1990; Zucker *et al.*, 1992).

Our studies also showed that the increase in the lipid motion (Δl) significantly raises as the pH drops from 8.0 to 7.4 and 7.0 (~3, ~6 and ~11 percent change, respectively, regarding carbon number 7 region), indicating that the membrane properties are further impaired by acidosis, and reinforcing the concept that uncharged diacid UCB is the molecular species involved in the UCB-induced disruption of cell integrity (Brito *et al.*, 2001).

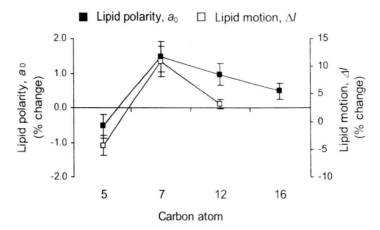

Figure 11. Unconjugated bilirubin impairs membrane dynamic properties of human erythrocyte membranes. Right-side-out vesicles were obtained from human erythrocytes of adult donors and were spin labeled with stearic acid molecules bearing a reporter group at different positions down the lipid chain, prior to incubation with either no addition (control) or 8.6 µM purified unconjugated bilirubin, for 15 min at pH 7.4, at 37°C. Alterations of the polarity environment and phospholipid motion were determined by electron paramagnetic resonance spectroscopy analysis, by measuring the isotropic hyperfine splitting constant (a0) and the outer half-width at half-height of the low field extremum (Δl), respectively. Statistically significant differences vs. respective control were obtained for both parameters; % changes were calculated based on corresponding controls. Derived from data of Brito et al. (2001).

Rat Brain Mitochondria

The UCB-induced perturbation of membrane dynamics has common features regardless the type of membrane model, as evidenced by the similar pattern of membrane dynamics perturbation observed in isolated rat brain mitochondria exposed to the pigment (Figure 12A). The results obtained using these organelles are consistent with the intercalation of UCB at C-5, rendering the inner regions more permeable and fluid, with the maximum effect achieved at C-7 (Rodrigues *et al.*, 2002c). The higher UCB concentrations required to induce the same magnitude of effects in erythrocytes may result either from a more generic perturbation or from the high plasticity of RBC.

The increased polarity of the mitochondrial membrane at the carbon number 7 region is also supported by the observation that UCB enhances the mobility of proteins (Figure 12B), indicating disruption of the protein order and increased membrane fluidity and permeability. Such membrane permeabilization is certainly involved in the UCB-induced cytochrome *c* release (Rodrigues *et al.*, 2000), which consequently leads to the disruption of the respiratory chain and redox status. This proposed model is corroborated by the fact that peroxidation of mitochondrial membrane lipids does indeed occur in these conditions (Figure 12B), despite the protective role of nanomolar concentrations of the pigment (Doré *et al.*, 1999; Mireles *et al.*, 2000).

So, taken together, these studies show that interaction of UCB with the mitochondrial membrane physically perturbs its structure, determining the disruption of lipid membrane polarity and fluidity and the alteration of protein order. The increased membrane permeability is consistent with the release of cytochrome c, leading to subsequent lipid peroxidation.

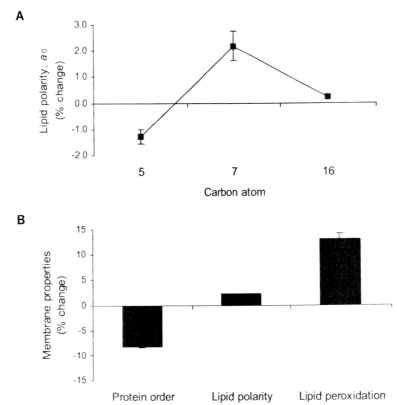

Figure 12. Unconjugated bilirubin disrupts membrane dynamic properties and redox status in rat brain mitochondria. Mitochondria were isolated from the brain of adult Wistar rats and were spin labeled prior to incubation with either no addition (control) or 4.3 μM purified unconjugated bilirubin, at pH 7.4, for 5 min at room temperature. Alterations of the polarity environment at different depths of the lipid chain were determined by electron paramagnetic resonance spectroscopy analysis, by measuring the isotropic hyperfine splitting constant (a_0) (A); modifications of the protein order and lipid polarity environment were determined using 4-maleimido-TEMPO and 7-doxyl stearic acid, respectively, while lipid peroxidation was evaluated using the 5-doxyl stearic acid spin label (B). Statistically significant differences vs. respective control were obtained for all the parameters; % changes were calculated based on corresponding controls. Derived from data of Rodrigues *et al.* (2002c).

Synaptosomal Membrane Systems

To ascertain whether UCB, at pathophysiologically relevant concentrations, also disturbs neuronal membranes, we pursuit our studies using synaptosomes, which are referred to mimic synaptic and neuronal functions *in vitro*, behaving as living neurons regarding respiration, oxygen uptake, maintenance of proper membrane potential, etc. (Whittaker, 1993). In this synaptosomal membrane system, UCB generates reactive oxygen species (ROS), which will lead to the protein oxidation and lipid peroxidation, also observed (Figure 13). These events are accompanied by a reduction in the GSH/GSSG ratio, reflecting an enhanced oxidation of GSH to GSSG and a reduced ability to restore GSH from GSSG, which must further contribute to the oxidative lesion of cell components.

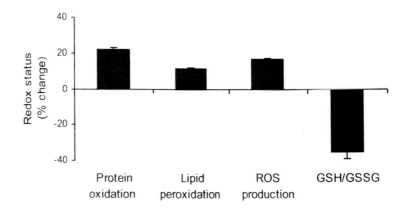

Figure 13. Unconjugated bilirubin disrupts the redox status in synaptosomal membrane systems. Synaptosomal vesicles were isolated from the brain cortex of Mongolian gerbils and incubated with either no addition (control) or 100 nM purified unconjugated bilirubin, at pH 7.4, for 4 h, at 37°C. Protein oxidation, lipid peroxidation, reactive oxygen species (ROS) production and disruption of glutathione metabolism were estimated by the measurement of protein carbonyls, production of 4-hydroxy-2-nonenal, oxidation of 2,7-dichlorofluorescein and enzymatic quantification of reduced (GSH) and oxidized (GSSG) glutathione, respectively. Statistically significant differences vs. respective control were obtained for all the parameters; % changes were calculated based on corresponding controls. Derived from data of Brito *et al.* (2004).

These modifications of the redox status are further accompanied by a disruption of the membrane assembly, evidenced by the redistribution of phosphatidylserine from the inner to the outer leaflet of the membrane (Figure 14), as previously observed in erythrocytes. To this loss of asymmetry must account, at least in part, the decreased activity of the aminophospholipid translocase. This translocase is a Mg^{2+}-ATPase also called flippase, responsible for the maintenance of phosphatidylserine in the inner leaflet of the membrane bilayer (Daleke and Lyles, 2000). In parallel, the activity of the Na^+,K^+-ATPase is also reduced, reflecting an overall impairment of membrane function by UCB. Such impairment presumably underlies the widespread dysfunction of the central nervous system by hyperbilirubinemia (Gourley, 1997). As a consequence, the sodium-calcium exchange system fails and a build-up of intrasynaptosomal calcium occurs. Since the maintenance of calcium homeostasis is crucial for neuron survival, the observed accumulation of intracellular calcium appears as a central event during UCB-induced neuronal death.

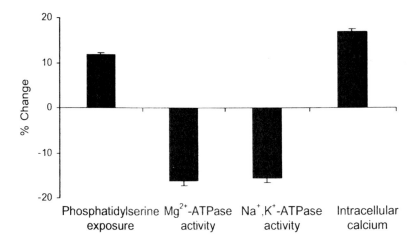

Figure 14. Unconjugated bilirubin disrupts membrane functionality, leading to loss of phospholipid asymmetry and calcium intrusion in synaptosomal membrane systems. Synaptosomal vesicles were isolated from Mongolian gerbils and incubated with either no addition (control) or 100 nM purified unconjugated bilirubin, at pH 7.4, for 4 h, at 37°C. Phosphatidylserine exposure and intracellular calcium were determined by the measurement of the fluorescence intensity of phosphatidylserine-bound annexin V and of the calcium chelator BAPTA-AM, respectively, while the activity of the membrane ATPases was estimated by evaluation of released phosphorus. Statistically significant differences vs. respective control were obtained for all the parameters; % changes were calculated based on corresponding controls. Derived from data of Brito *et al.* (2004).

Taken collectively, the results of this study establish a link between hyperbilirubinemia, oxidative stress and injury to neocortical synaptosomes (Brito *et al.*, 2004), and lead to the proposal of a model where oxidative stress appears as a key player in the pathways of neuronal damage by UCB (Figure 15). According to this model, UCB promotes oxidative stress in synaptosomal membrane systems, by means of ROS formation, protein oxidation and lipid peroxidation, to which further contributes the disruption of the protective role played by glutathione metabolism. Thus, crucial aspects of cell function are impaired, such as the activity of the flippase. As a result, the bilayer asymmetry is disrupted and phosphatidylserine is exposed at the outer leaflet of the membrane bilayer, favoring the recognition and removal of dying cells. To the loss of the asymmetric distribution of phospholipids shall also concur the oxidation of phosphatidylserine by direct ROS attack. The reduced activity of the Na^+,K^--ATPase, not only reflects the impairment of membrane function by UCB, but also leads to intracellular calcium overload, further enhancing ROS formation and adding to oxidative injury. In turn, accumulation of intracellular calcium can conceivably be responsible for the fall in the rate at which phosphatidylserine is translocated, and contribute to further reduce Na^-,K^--ATPase activity, which requires normal concentrations of calcium, as well as of the negatively charged phospholipid for normal activity (Lees, 1991).

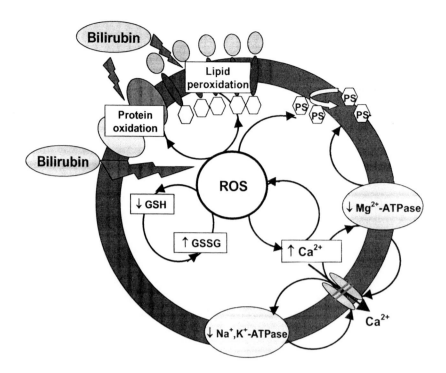

Figure 15. Simplified model establishing the relevance of oxidative stress in the pathways of neuronal damage by unconjugated bilirubin. Unconjugated bilirubin, at pathophysiologically relevant concentrations, promotes oxidative stress in synaptosomal membrane systems, by means of reactive oxygen species (ROS) formation, protein oxidation and lipid peroxidation, together with the impaired ability to restore reduced glutathione (GSH) from the oxidized one (GSSG). Consequently, the activity of the aminophospholipid translocase, a Mg^{2+}-ATPase, is reduced, resulting in the exposure of phosphatidylserine (PS) at the outer leaflet of the membrane bilayer, and disruption of bilayer asymmetry. To this fact shall also contribute the oxidation of PS by direct ROS attack. The activity of the Na^+,K^+-ATPase is also reduced, promoting intracellular calcium overload, which further enhances ROS formation, adding to oxidative injury. In turn, accumulation of intracellular calcium can be responsible for the fall in the rate at which PS is translocated, contributing to a further reduction of Na^+,K^+-ATPase activity, and overall impairment of membrane function by unconjugated bilirubin.

UNCONJUGATED BILIRUBIN DISRUPTS MEMBRANE PROPERTIES OF INTACT BRAIN CELLS AND CAUSES NERVE CELL DEATH

Unconjugated Bilirubin Toxicity Involves Alterations of Glutamate Transport and Secretion

The amino acid glutamate is a small-molecule neurotransmitter, generally recognized as the most important excitatory transmitter for the normal function of the brain. The great majority of excitatory neurons in the central nervous system is glutamatergic, and over half of all brain synapses release this molecule (Meldrum, 2000; Savolainen *et al.*, 1996). Glutamate is removed from the synaptic cleft by specific membrane transporters, mainly present in astrocyte brain population. If transport fails, over activation of neuronal glutamate receptors engenders neurodegeneration by a mechanism known as excitotoxicity involving, at least in part, mitochondrial damage (Meldrum, 2000; Schinder *et al.*, 1996; Stout *et al.*, 1998).

An association between excitotoxic damage and jaundice was first verified by McDonald *et al.* (1998) who found that administration of the glutamate agonist (NMDA) to Gunn rat pups (a jaundiced rat species) leads to increased injury, and that simultaneous treatment with a glutamate receptor antagonist reduces the lesion size. Our own studies, have demonstrated that the uptake of glutamate by astrocytes is greatly reduced by UCB (Figure 16), and follows a time- and concentration-dependent profile, which is already significant by 5 min interaction with the pigment (Silva *et al.*, 1999). A lower, but still significant, inhibition is also observed when cortical neurons in primary culture are exposed to UCB (Silva et al., 2002). More recently, we showed that UCB not only impairs the neurotransmitter uptake but also induces its release from exposed cells (Falcão *et al.*, 2004, 2005), as indicated in Figure 16. Like the uptake inhibition, glutamate release is also very fast and statistically relevant after 5 min exposure (Silva *et al.*, 2004). It is then conceivable that UCB exerts its neurotoxic action, at least in part, by engendering or aggravating the excitotoxic injury. These studies further point out that, during UCB encephalopathy, neurons are not the only targets and that other brain cells, like astrocytes, may play a key role in neurodegeneration.

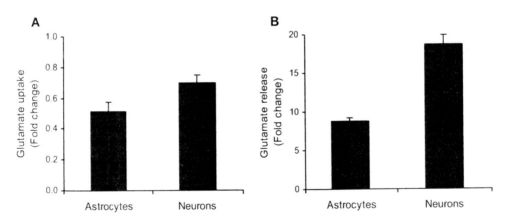

Figure 16. Unconjugated bilirubin inhibits glutamate uptake and induces its release in primary cultures of astrocytes and neurons. Rat cortical astrocytes or neurons were incubated with either no addition (control) or 100 μM purified unconjugated bilirubin, plus 100 μM human serum albumin, at pH 7.4, for 15 min (A) or 4 h (B), at 37°C. Glutamate uptake was measured by scintillation count in cell lysates following 7 min incubation with [³H]glutamate (A); secretion of glutamate was determined enzymatically (B). Statistically significant differences vs. respective control were obtained for both parameters; fold changes were calculated based on corresponding controls. Derived from data of Silva et al. (2002), and Falcão et al. (2004, 2005).

Endocytosis is Impaired in Unconjugated Bilirubin-treated Cells

Alterations in membrane functions of brain cells by UCB are not restricted to impairment of neurotransmitter transport or excessive secretion of glutamate. Using again astrocytes as a model, we demonstrated that endocytosis, a crucial vital function of those glial cells, is greatly reduced by exposure to UCB (Silva *et al.*, 2001a). It is established that cationized ferritin (CF) binds to anionic sites on cell membranes and is progressively internalized to endocytic compartments (Lindo *et al.*, 1993). This normal pathway is rapidly (15 min) disrupted by UCB (171 µM, UCB/HSA molar ratio of 3), reducing not only the intracellular accumulation of CF but also its membrane binding (Figure 17). Moreover, such effects seem to be independent from cytoskeletal alterations, once they are only observed at a latter time (4 h) and for the highest UCB level (Silva *et al.*, 2001a). In addition, morphological alterations of the rough endoplasmic reticulum and mitochondria can also be observed.

Another piece of evidence regarding UCB alterations of cell function can be added by the use of MTT, which conversion to formazan reflects the cellular metabolic performance. In fact, MTT seems to be taken up by endocytosis and, following reduction, excreted by exocytosis (Liu et al., 1997). Therefore, a low reduction level must correspond to an impaired cell function. In our studies, we found that neurons exposed to 86 µM UCB (UCB to HSA molar ratio of 3) exhibit a 60% reduction in MTT metabolization. In the same conditions, astrocytes were even more affected by UCB, displaying a 70% decrease in MTT reduction

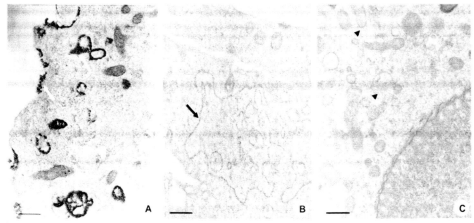

(Silva et al., 2002).

Figure 17. Unconjugated bilirubin inhibits cationized ferritin (CF) endocytosis in cultured astrocytes. Rat cortical astrocytes were incubated with either no addition (A) or 171 µM purified unconjugated bilirubin (UCB) (B,C), plus 57 µM human serum albumin, at pH 7.4, for 15 min, at 37°C. Following incubation, cells were treated with CF for 30 min, fixed and processed for transmission electron microscopy. UCB reduces CF labeling (white arrow), while induces the enlargement of the rough endoplasmic reticulum (black arrow) and the appearance of abnormal mitochondria morphology (arrowheads). Bar: 0.5 µm.

Taken together, these data reinforce the concept that cell membranes are important targets of UCB cytotoxicity. Furthermore, it is now apparent that UCB, besides membranes, has multiple targets and affects different cells in the brain. It is also interesting to notice that astrocytes seem to be functionally more affected than neurons following UCB exposure, suggesting again more than one course of action during UCB cytotoxicity.

Unconjugated Bilirubin Causes Dual Features of Cell Death in Nerve Cells

Given the extensive structural and functional alterations induced by UCB previously described, we can anticipate that nerve cells are necrotically killed when exposed to UCB. So, it is not surprising that UCB (86 μM; UCB/HSA molar ratio of 3) causes a time-dependent decrease of astrocyte viability (Silva et al., 2001b), assessed by trypan blue dye exclusion, a marker for necrosis. In fact, the loss of cell viability is already significant at 4 h exposure (P<0.01) and is sharply aggravated from 8 to 24 h (Figure 18A).

The release of LDH to the incubation medium by cells with a disrupted membrane is also a characteristic feature of necrosis. As expected, a 4 h exposure to 86 μM UCB causes approximately a 10% increase in LDH release (2.5-fold over control values) by astrocytes (Silva et al., 2002). In contrast with the outcome on glutamate uptake and MTT metabolization, it is interesting to observe that exposing neurons to the same incubation conditions previously described for astrocytes, causes the necrotic death of approximately 30% of neuronal cells (5-fold over control values), an effect 2–times greater than the one observed for glial cells (Figure 18B). This increased susceptibility to cell death found in our culture model system was also described for neuroblastoma versus glioblastoma or astrocytoma cell lines (Ngai et al., 2000; Notter and Kendig, 1986).

Alterations on mitochondrial function and permeability, together with increased production of ROS and the release of caspase activators have been associated with the onset of apoptotic cell death (Green and Reed, 1998; Kroemer et al., 1998). As previously described, UCB also affects mitochondria and disrupts the redox status; so, evaluating the participation of this death mechanism in UCB neurological damage grew in importance. In fact, as for necrosis, astrocytes display a time-dependent sensitivity to UCB concerning apoptosis (Figure 18A), assessed by relative quantification of fragmented nuclei. UCB-induced apoptosis at 4 h incubation (86 μM) was approximately 14%, a value which is at the same level of magnitude of that obtained for cell death by necrosis (Silva et al., 2001b).

Cell death by apoptosis was also differently demonstrated by astrocytes and neurons (Silva et al., 2002). Similarly to necrosis, when incubated with the same UCB concentration, apoptotic death of neurons was ~5-fold over control values (corresponding to 24% UCB-induced apoptosis) and superior to that of astrocytes (~4-fold over controls) (Figure 18B). So, it seems clear that, at least in the selected experimental conditions, neurons are in fact more prone to an irreversible injury by UCB than astrocytes. Again, these results suggest that UCB toxicity to brain cells is promoted by more than one mechanism, depending of the cell type, which can lead to either reversible or irreversible injury, being the neurons apparently more vulnerable to permanent lesion. Time-dependent induced cytotoxicity and apoptosis was also observed when astrocytes were exposed to serum obtained from hyperbilirubinemic newborns, reinforcing the involvement of this feature in UCB neurotoxic damage (Kumral et al., 2005). The participation of both necrotic and apoptotic mechanisms in nerve cell death seems to vary according to time of exposure and pigment concentration, with a severe stress preferably resulting in increased necrosis and a moderate exposure rather leading to apoptosis. This is consistent with data obtained in a human teratocarcinoma-derived neuronal cell line, where UCB was shown to induce necrosis at high and moderate concentration even in shorter incubation periods, and apoptosis was predominant for lower induction levels at latter periods (Hankø et al., 2005).

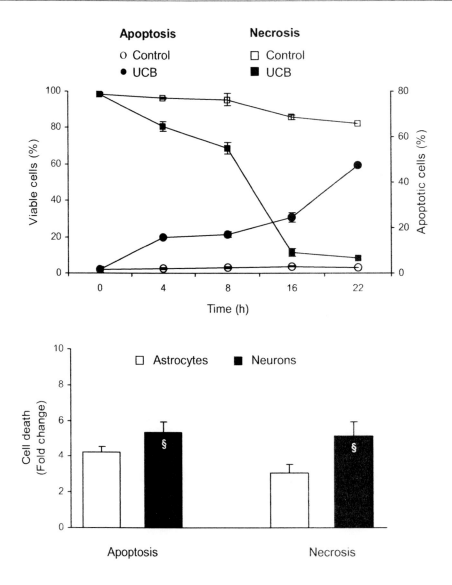

Figure 18. Unconjugated bilirubin causes cell death both by apoptosis and necrosis in primary cultures of astrocytes and neurons. Rat cortical astrocytes or neurons were incubated with either no addition (control) or 86 µM purified unconjugated bilirubin (UCB), plus 29 µM human serum albumin, at pH 7.4, at 37°C. Astrocytes were exposed to UCB for different time points, and apoptosis was assessed by nuclear morphological changes after Hoechst staining, while viable cells were scored by trypan blue dye exclusion (A). Both astrocytes and neurons were incubated for 4 h and apoptosis was assessed by the TUNEL assay while necrosis was measured by means of the release of LDH by nonviable cells (B). Statistically significant differences vs. respective control were obtained for both parameters; §P<0.01 from astrocytes. Derived from data of Silva *et al.* (2001b, 2002).

UCB-induced apoptosis is not restricted to neurons and astrocytes. Recent reports have shown that other brain cells like oligodendrocytes (Genc *et al.*, 2003) or endothelial cell (Akin *et al.*, 2002) also display dual features of cell death, both necrosis and apoptosis. Moreover, apoptosis is not constrained to brain cells since hepatoma cell lines (Seubert *et al.*,

2002) and colon cancer cells (Keshavan *et al.*, 2004) when exposed to UCB also die by an apoptotic mechanism, that seems to involve caspase-3 activation and mitochondrial cytochrome *c* release. Accordingly, we found that cytochrome *c* release through mitochondrial membrane permeabilization is as well implicated in the apoptosis of astrocytes and neurons following UCB incubation (Rodrigues *et al.*, 2000). At least in neurons, this apoptotic mechanism involves Bax translocation to mitochondria, caspase-3 activation and PARP degradation, reinforcing the concept that the mitochondrial pathway is an important contributor to UCB-induced nerve cell apoptosis (Rodrigues *et al.*, 2002b). Activation by UCB of the cell surface death receptor, tumor necrosis factor receptor 1 (TNFR1), leading to activation of mitogen-activated protein kinases (MAPKs) (Fernandes *et al.*, 2006; Lin *et al.*, 2003), suggests that the extrinsic apoptotic pathway is also involved (Figure 19).

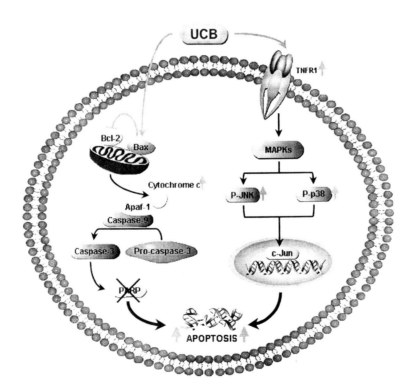

Figure 19. Schematic representation of unconjugated bilirubin-induced apoptosis via the intrinsic (mitochondrial) pathway and extrinsic (TNFR1) pathway. Treatment of nerve cells with purified unconjugated bilirubin (UCB) leads to the release of cytochrome *c*. At the same time, translocation of Bax to the mitochondrial membrane might inactivate Bcl-2 and originate the formation of selective ion pores in membranes, further contributing to the release of cytochrome *c*. In cytosol, cytochrome *c* binds to the apoptosis protease activating factor-1 (Apaf-1), triggering the activation of caspase 9. Caspase 9 cleaves and activates pro-caspase-3 to its active form, which results in the PARP degradation and execution of the cell-death programme (mitochondrial pathway). UCB also activates the cell surface death receptor, tumor necrosis factor receptor 1 (TNFR1), leading to activation of the mitogen-activated protein kinases (MAPKs), Jun N-terminal kinase (JNK) and p38, to the phosphorylated forms (P-JNK and P-p38), which can promote apoptosis via the c-Jun transcription factor (extrinsic pathway).

Unconjugated Bilirubin Differently Affects the Redox Status of Neurons and Astrocytes

Despite the UCB ability to damage both neurons and astrocytes, the different response of these cellular types point to distinct pathways of neurotoxicity, where oxidative injury emerges as a key player. In fact, our newest data show that UCB promotes protein oxidation and lipid peroxidation in neurons (Figure 20), while astrocytes are less susceptible to oxidative damage of membrane components (data not shown). This finding is not without precedent, since other studies have reported that astrocytes are more resistant to oxidative injury than neurons (Almeida *et al.*, 2002; Bolaños *et al.*, 1995; Schmuck *et al.*, 2002). To this fact, shall primarily account the greater antioxidant defense mechanisms of astrocytes, such as the increased intracellular content of GSH (Dringen *et al.*, 2000), as well as the higher levels and response of their antioxidant enzymes (Makar *et al.*, 1994; Schmuck *et al.*, 2002). Nevertheless, our results also reveal that UCB induces a statistically significant production of ROS in astrocytes, though the increment over control values is remarkably inferior to that observed in neurons (Figure 20). The generation of ROS herewith observed by fluorescence microscopy validates our previous EPR spectroscopy analysis (Figure 12B), where a loss of paramagnetism of a spin-labeled probe reported the production of free radicals (Rodrigues *et al.*, 2002a). On the other hand, the higher extent of ROS production in neurons is corroborated by previous observations regarding the neurotoxin paraquat (Schmuck *et al.*, 2002). Therefore, it is conceivable that as ROS are generated by UCB interaction, the antioxidant defenses are able to promote their reduction, thus decreasing or preventing the oxidation of membrane components to occur in astrocytes, but not in neurons. Moreover, astrocytes are resistant to oxidative injury, even in the presence of an aggravating condition such as endotoxin (data not shown), despite the ability of this toxin to augment the UCB-induced secretion of pro-inflammatory cytokines and cell death presented below.

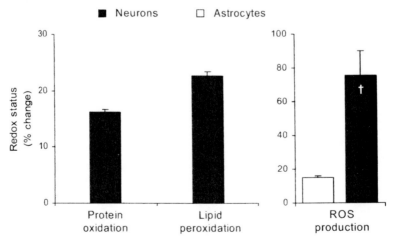

Figure 20. Unconjugated bilirubin disrupts the redox status of nerve cells. Rat cortical neurons or astrocytes were incubated with either no addition (control) or 100 nM purified unconjugated bilirubin, at pH 7.4, for 4 h, at 37°C. Protein oxidation, lipid peroxidation and reactive oxygen species (ROS) production were estimated by the measurement of protein carbonyls, 4-hydroxy-2-nonenal and oxidation of dihydrorhodamine, respectively. Statistically significant differences vs. respective control were obtained for all the parameters; % changes were calculated based on corresponding controls. [†]P<0.05 from astrocytes.

FACTORS AND CONDITIONS THAT MAY AGGRAVATE UNCONJUGATED BILIRUBIN NEUROTOXICITY

There is evidence that the serum UCB concentration does not provide a reliable estimate of its production, the tissue concentrations achieved, or the albumin-bound UCB levels. Moreover, a correlation between the serum UCB concentration and encephalopathy has never been conclusively established (Blanckaert and Fevery, 1990; Dennery et al., 2001; Gourley, 1997; Kaplan and Hammerman, 2004; Reiser, 2004). This fact seems to result from the presence of several risk factors, which can aggravate sequelae due to UCB encephalopathy (Hansen, 2002). Among such factors, the roles of the time of exposure, infection and prematurity still remain under-explained or controversial.

Time of Exposure

It has been suggested that the duration of hyperbilirubinemia, in addition to the peak serum UCB levels, is an important determinant of the pigment concentration in the brain. Therefore, the time of exposure to UCB appears to play a key role in UCB encephalopathy and in the impairment of long-term neurologic development (Blanckaert and Fevery, 1990; Dennery et al., 2001; Gourley, 1997; Kaplan and Hammerman, 2004; Reiser, 2004). So, we evaluated the extent of cell death as a function of the incubation period using more clinically relevant conditions (UCB/HSA molar ratio of 1) in an attempt to establish the influence of the length of hyperbilirubinemia on the neurotoxic effects of UCB. Our studies showed that the LDH release by non viable cells increase along the time of exposure (Figure 21), reaching levels of cell death higher than 40% by 24 h exposure of astrocytes to the pigment (Fernandes et al., 2005). These results highlight the relevance of the timing of cell exposure to the pigment on the UCB-induced neurotoxicity, and provide a basis for the increasingly development of neurologic abnormalities in children exposed to UCB (>20 mg/dL) for less than 6 h or for more than 12 h (Blanckaert and Fevery, 1990; Dennery et al., 2001; Gourley, 1997; Kaplan and Hammerman, 2004; Reiser, 2004).

Sepsis and Inflammation

Lipopolysaccharide (LPS) from Escherichia coli is an endotoxin that has been used in association with UCB to mimic septic conditions during hyperbilirubinemia, both in vivo (Allen et al., 1998; Hansen et al., 1993) and in vitro (Ngai and Yeung, 1999; Yeung and Ngai, 2001), but so far the experimental data do not fully explain the clinical evidence of aggravated UCB encephalopathy during sepsis.

Our results showed that LPS increases the extent of UCB-induced cell death by necrosis in astrocyte cultures (Fernandes *et al.*, 2004b), which is in agreement with the decreased viability observed in fibroblasts (Ngai and Yeung, 1999; Yeung and Ngai, 2001) and endothelial cells (Ngai and Yeung, 1999; Yeung and Ngai, 2001). Furthermore, LPS concentrations as low as 1 and 10 ng/mL immunostimulates cultured astrocytes, leading to the significant production of tumor necrosis factor-α (TNF-α) and interleukin (IL)-6, although with a lower effect on IL-1β secretion (Fernandes *et al.*, 2004b). It was very interesting and quite unexpected to notice that UCB itself has immunostimulant properties on astrocyte cultures (Figure 22). To exclude an eventual participation of cell death we used incubation conditions (UCB/HSA molar ratio of 0.5, for 4 h) where both apoptosis and necrosis are inferior to 10%. In these conditions, UCB has an equivalent effect to LPS regarding TNF-α secretion, and a higher capacity to induce IL-1β production.

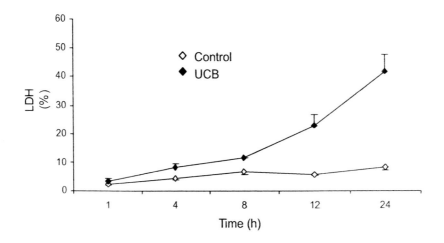

Figure 21. The time of exposure enhances the extent of cell death induced by unconjugated bilirubin. Rat cortical astrocytes were incubated with either no addition (control) or 100 µM purified unconjugated bilirubin (UCB), in the presence of 100 µM human serum albumin, at pH 7.4, for different time points, at 37°C. Cell death by necrosis was estimated by the measurement of LDH release by nonviable cells. Significant differences (P<0.01) vs. respective control were obtained for all the time points except 1 h. Derived from data of Fernandes *et al.* (2005).

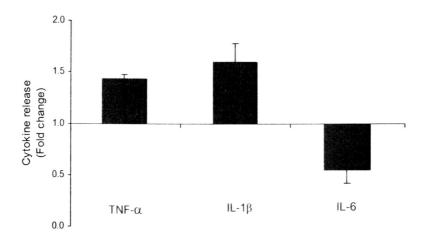

Figure 22. Unconjugated bilirubin modulates the production of cytokines by astrocytes. Rat cortical astrocytes were incubated with either no addition (control) or 50 μM purified unconjugated bilirubin (UCB), plus 100 μM human serum albumin, at pH 7.4, for 4 h, at 37°C. Cytokines released to the incubation media were assessed by ELISA. Statistically significant differences were obtained for all the parameters vs. respective control. Derived from data of Fernandes *et al.* (2004b).

Conversely, while LPS stimulates the release of IL-6, UCB causes a marked decrease of the extracellular levels of this interleukin by 4 h exposure. Co-incubation with LPS further increases the UCB-induced production of the pro-inflammatory cytokines TNF-α and IL-1β, but does not modify IL-6 decrease (Figure 23). Notably, LPS has no effect on UCB-induced release of glutamate, indicating that the inflammatory mechanism can be independent from the membrane actions of UCB, and reinforcing once more the involvement of multiple mechanisms in UCB-nerve cell interaction. UCB-induced cytokine release seems to involve NF-κB activation via TNFR1 signaling (Fernandes *et al.*, 2004a, 2006; Lin *et al.*, 2003), which in part is consistent with the participation of the apoptosis extrinsic pathway already suggested (Figure 19). These results reveal the involvement of inflammation during hyperbilirubinemic encephalopathy and may substantiate the observed exacerbation of this condition when associated with sepsis.

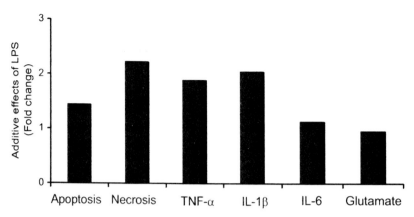

Figure 23. Lipopolysaccharide potentiates the injurious and immunostimulatory properties of unconjugated bilirubin in astrocytes, but not the release of glutamate. Rat cortical astrocytes were incubated with either no addition (control), 50 μM purified unconjugated bilirubin (UCB), or a combination of UCB and 1 ng/mL lipopolysaccharide (LPS), in the presence of 100 μM human serum albumin, at pH 7.4, for 4 h, at 37°C. Apoptosis was assessed by nuclear morphological changes after Hoechst staining and necrosis by means of the release of LDH by nonviable cells. Cytokines and glutamate released to the incubation media were assessed by ELISA and by an enzymatic assay, respectively. Statistically significant differences were obtained for all the parameters between UCB-treated samples and respective controls. Fold changes were calculated between UCB plus LPS and UCB alone-treated groups, and significant differences (P<0.05) were obtained for cell death by necrosis, and secretion of TNF-α and IL-1β. Derived from data of Fernandes *et al.* (2004b).

Cell Differentiation

As stated above, prematurity is also considered a risk factor for neurotoxicity during neonatal hyperbilirubinemia. There is current opinion that immaturity is associated with a greater sensitivity to neuronal sequelae of UCB. In fact, studies performed by us (Rodrigues *et al.*, 2002d) and others (Rhine *et al.*, 1999) in nerve cell culture models point out that UCB is more cytotoxic, i.e. produces greater cell death, in more immature cells than in older cultures. In fact, we have demonstrated that astrocytes cultured for 5 days *in vitro* (DIV), as well as 4 DIV neurons exposed to 86 μM UCB (UCB/HSA molar ratio of 3) reveal approximately 2-fold higher levels of apoptosis and necrosis, when compared to 10 and 8 DIV astrocytes and neurons, respectively (Rodrigues *et al.*, 2002d). In agreement, the pro-inflammatory response, the release of glutamate and the extent of cell death due to UCB interaction are higher in undifferentiated astrocytes (5 DIV) (Figure 24) and decrease with age-in-culture (Falcão *et al.*, 2005). Ongoing studies also suggest that, regarding the inflammatory response, cultured neurons display the same age-dependent pattern as astrocytes, although the absolute levels of secreted cytokines and glutamate are markedly inferior (Falcão *et al.*, 2004). These results are a start up point for the research that, hopefully, will generate a better understanding of the proneness of premature infants to bilirubin encephalopathy.

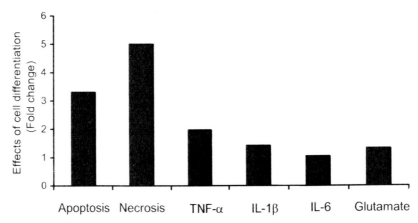

Figure 24 Undifferentiated astrocytes are more prone to damage by unconjugated bilirubin than more mature cells. Rat cortical astrocytes, cultured *in vitro* for 5 or 20 days, were incubated with either no addition (control) or 50 μM purified unconjugated bilirubin, plus 100 μM human serum albumin, at pH 7.4, for 4 h, at 37°C. Apoptosis was assessed by nuclear morphological changes after Hoechst staining and necrosis by the release of LDH by nonviable cells. Cytokines and glutamate released to the incubation media were assessed by ELISA and by an enzymatic assay, respectively. Significant differences (P<0.01) were obtained for all the parameters vs. respective control; fold changes were calculated between 5 and 20 days *in vitro* astrocytes exposed to unconjugated bilirubin. Derived from data of Falcão *et al.* (2005).

CONCLUSION

Although free UCB levels below the aqueous saturation limit appear to protect cells against oxidative damage, above the 70 nM threshold this protection is lost because of the countervailing toxicity of high concentrations of the pigment. The fact that toxic effects start to appear at concentrations near or above the aqueous solubility limit, where UCB monomers, soluble oligomers and metastable small colloids are likely to be present, renders untenable the long-accepted concept that marked supersaturation and precipitation of UCB are necessary to produce neurotoxicity (Brodersen and Stern, 1990). Monomers of UCB diacid intercalate superficially in the hydrocarbon core of the membrane bilayer and the resultant modest perturbation of membrane structure appears as a factor in the early cellular toxicity of clinically relevant concentrations of UCB.

Cells exposed to UCB suffer complex alterations in a variety of vital cell functions, leading to cell death with mixed features of apoptosis and necrosis. Despite the UCB ability to damage both neurons and astrocytes, the different response of these cellular types point to distinct pathways of neurotoxicity, where oxidative injury emerges as a key factor. Whatever the mechanisms, development of UCB cytotoxicity is determined by free UCB levels and is aggravated by acidosis and sepsis. In addition, fetal cells bind UCB more avidly and show early signs of decreased viability, appearing as sensitive targets for UCB toxicity. These findings, together with the enhanced inflammatory response by immature nerve cells, provide a basis for prematurity as a risk factor for kernicterus.

In conclusion, through this journey along the complex alterations in a variety of cell functions, some of the key molecular events and mediators during hyperbilirubinemia are clarified, providing insights into the mechanisms of brain damage by UCB, essential to improve the risk assessment. Nevertheless, further studies are needed to discriminate between cell membrane and mitochondria as the primary target of UCB neurotoxicity. We must also keep in mind that UCB has dual effects, possessing strong antioxidant properties at low levels while at high concentrations it increases intracellular ROS production and cytotoxicity. However, it is still necessary to clearly differentiate the UCB level responsible for biologically relevant effects from that inducing cell damage. Finally, additional studies are also required to clarify the cascade of events and mediators intervening in UCB-induced acute neuronal dysfunction and long-term adverse neurodevelopmental effects. The dissection of the molecular mechanisms involved in UCB neurotoxicity may yield new targets upon which to focus drug discovery efforts aimed at reducing brain injury and disabilities by UCB.

ACKNOWLEDGEMENTS

The Authors wish to express their appreciation to all the co-Authors of the publications which findings are described in this review, in particular, Adelaide Fernandes, Ana Sofia Falcão, Deolinda Matos, Cecília Rodrigues, José Moura, Lucinda Mata, Sérgio Gulbenkian, Allan Butterfield and Claudio Tiribelli. Studies from the Authors' Research Unit were funded by Fundação para a Ciência e a Tecnologia (Portugal).

REFERENCES

Akin, E.; Clower, B.; Tibbs, R.; Tang, J. & Zhang, J. (2002). Bilirubin produces apoptosis in cultured bovine brain endothelial cells. *Brain Res, 931*, 168-175.

Allen, J. W.; Tommarello, S.; Carcillo, J. & Hansen, T. W. (1998). Effects of endotoxemia and sepsis on bilirubin oxidation by rat brain mitochondrial membranes. *Biol Neonate, 73*, 340-345.

Almeida, A.; Delgado-Esteban, M.; Bolaños, J. P. & Medina, J. M. (2002). Oxygen and glucose deprivation induces mitochondrial dysfunction and oxidative stress in neurones but not in astrocytes in primary culture. *J Neurochem, 81*, 207-217.

American Academy of Pediatrics (2004). Management of hyperbilirubinemia in the newborn infant 35 or more weeks of gestation. *Pediatrics, 114*, 297-316.

Barañano, D. E.; Rao, M.; Ferris, C. D. & Snyder, S. H. (2002). Biliverdin reductase: a major physiologic cytoprotectant. *Proc Natl Acad Sci U S A, 99*, 16093-16098.

Barthez, J. P.; Boisseau, C.; Bentata, J. & Borderon, E. (1986). Étude de la bilirubine érythrocytaire. Appréciation du risque d'ictère nucléaire. *Pathol Biol, 30*, 252-256.

Bennett, V. (1985). The membrane skeleton of human erythrocytes and its implications for more complex cells. *Ann Rev Biochem, 54*, 273-304.

Berk, P. D. & Noyer, C. (1994). Bilirubin metabolism and the hereditary hyperbilirubinemias. *Semin Liver Dis, 14*, 325-345.

Blanckaert, N. & Fevery, J. (1990) Physiology and pathology of bilirubin metabolism. *Hepatology. A textbook of liver disease*, Vol.1, pp. 254-303. Zakim, D.; Boyer, T. D. Eds., Philadelphia, WB Saunders Company.

Bolaños, J. P.; Heales, S. J.; Land, J. M. & Clark, J. B. (1995). Effect of peroxynitrite on the mitochondrial respiratory chain: differential susceptibility of neurones and astrocytes in primary culture. *J Neurochem, 64*, 1965-1972.

Bouillerot, A.; Fessard, C. & Sauger, F. (1981). La bilirubine érythrocytaire: ses variations - interêt pratique de son dosage. *Clin Chim Acta, 109*, 39-44.

Bratlid, D. (1972). The effect of pH on bilirubin binding to human erythrocytes. *Scand J Clin Lab Invest, 29*, 453-459.

Brites, D.; Brito, A. & Silva, R. (1997). Effect of bilirubin on erythrocyte shape and haemolysis, under hypotonic, aggregating or non-aggregating conditions, and correlation with cell age. *Scand J Clin Lab Invest, 57*, 337-350.

Brito, A.; Silva, R. F. & Brites, D. (2002). Bilirubin induces loss of membrane lipids and exposure of phosphatidylserine in human erythrocytes. *Cell Biol Toxicol, 18*, 181-192.

Brito, M. A. (2001). Interacção da bilirrubina com a membrana do eritrócito. Espécies moleculares envolvidas, estádios de toxicidade e comportamento da célula fetal. *PhD Thesis*, University of Lisbon.

Brito, M. A. & Brites, D. (2003). Effect of acidosis on bilirubin-induced toxicity to human erythrocytes. *Mol Cell Biochem, 247*, 155-162.

Brito, M. A.; Brites, D. & Butterfield, D. A. (2004). A link between hyperbilirubinemia, oxidative stress and injury to neocortical synaptosomes. *Brain Res, 1026*, 33-43.

Brito, M. A.; Brondino, C. D.; Moura, J. J. G. & Brites, D. (2001). Effects of bilirubin molecular species on membrane dynamic properties of human erythrocyte membranes: a spin label electron paramagnetic resonance spectroscopy study. *Arch Biochem Biophys, 387*, 57-65.

Brito, M. A.; Silva, R.; Matos, D. C.; Silva, A. T. & Brites, D. (1996). Alterations of erythrocyte morphology and lipid composition by hyperbilirubinemia. *Clin Chim Acta, 249*, 149-165.

Brito, M. A.; Silva, R.; Tiribelli, C. & Brites, D. (2000). Assessment of bilirubin toxicity to erythrocytes. Implication in neonatal jaundice management. *Eur J Clin Invest, 30*, 239-247.

Brodersen, R. (1981) Binding of bilirubin to albumin and tissues. *Phsysiological and Biochemical Basis for Perinatal Medicine.* Samuel Z. Levine Conference, First International Meeting, Paris, 1979, pp. 144-152. Monset-Couchard, M.; Minkowski, A. Eds., Basel, S. Karger.

Brodersen, R. (1979). Bilirubin. Solubility and interaction with albumin and phospholipid. *J Biol Chem, 254*, 2364-2369.

Brodersen, R. & Stern, L. (1990). Deposition of bilirubin acid in the central nervous system – a hypothesis for the development of kernicterus. *Acta Paediatr Scand, 79*, 12-19.

Cashore, W. J. (1980). Free bilirubin concentrations and bilirubin-binding affinity in term and preterm infants. *J Pediatr, 96*, 521-527.

Cestaro, B.; Cervato, G.; Ferrari, S.; Di Silvestro, G.; Monti, D. & Manitto, P. (1983). Interaction of bilirubin with small unilamellar vesicles of dipalmitoylphosphatidylcholine. *Ital J Biochem, 32*, 318-329.

Clark, J. E.; Foresti, R.; Green, C. J. & Motterlini, R. (2000). Dynamics of haem oxygenase-1 expression and bilirubin production in cellular protection against oxidative stress. *Biochem J, 3483*, 615-619.

Daleke, D. L. & Lyles, J. V. (2000). Identification and purification of aminophospholipid flippases. *Biochim Biophys Acta, 1486*, 108-127.

Day, L. (1954). Inhibition of brain respiration in vitro by bilirubin: reversal of inhibition by various means. *Am J Dis Child, 88*, 504-506.

Dennery, P. A.; Seidman, D. S. & Stevenson, D. K. (2001). Neonatal hyperbilirubienmia. *N Eng J Med, 344*, 581-590.

Doré, S.; Goto, S.; Sampei, K.; Blackshaw, S.; Hester, L. D.; Ingi, T.; Sawa, A.; Traystman, R. J.; Koehler, R. C. & Snyder, S. H. (2000). Heme oxygenase-2 acts to prevent neuronal death in brain cultures and following transient cerebral ischemia. *Neuroscience, 99*, 587-592.

Doré, S.; Takahashi, M.; Ferris, C. D.; Hester, L. D.; Guastella, D. & Snyder, S. H. (1999). Bilirubin, formed by activation of heme oxygenase-2, protects neurons against oxidative stress injury. *Proc Natl Acad Sci, 96*, 2445-2450.

Dringen, R.; Gutterer, J. M. & Hirrlinger, J. (2000). Glutathione metabolism in brain. Metabolic interaction between astrocytes and neurons in the defense against reactive oxygen species. *Eur J Biochem, 267*, 4912-4916.

Ebbesen, F. (2000). Recurrence of kernicterus in term and near-term infants in Denmark. *Acta Paediatr, 89*, 1213-1217.

Ernster, L. & Zetterström, R. (1956). Bilirubin, an uncoupler of oxidative phosphorylation in isolated mitochondria. *Nature, 178*, 1335-1337.

Falcão, A. S.; Fernandes, A,. Brito, M. A,. Silva, R. F. & Brites, D. (2004). Bilirubin-induced release of cytokines and glutamate depends from neural cell type and decreases with differentiation. *Pediatr. Res., 55, [4, Part 2]*, 474A.

Falcão, A. S.; Fernandes, A.; Brito, M. A.; Silva, R. F. M. & Brites, D. (2005). Bilirubin-induced inflammatory response, glutamate release, and cell death in rat cortical astrocytes are enhanced in younger cells. *Neurobiol. Dis., 20*, 199-206.

Fernandes, A., Falcão, A. S.; Gordo, C.; Gama, M. J.; Silva, R. F. M.; Brito, M. A. & Brites, D. (2005). Dissecting astrocyte reactivity by unconjugated bilirubin: evidence for a biphasic response. *2005 Pediatric Academic Societies' Annual Meeting*, 1944A.

Fernandes, A., Falcão, A. S., Silva, R. F. M.; Gordo, A. C.; Gama, M. J.; Brito, M. A. & Brites, D. (2006). Inflammatory signaling pathways involved in astroglial activation by bilirubin. *J. Neurochem. (in press)*.

Fernandes, A.; Falcão, A. S.; Silva, R. F.; Brito, M. A. & Brites, D. (2004a). Role of TNF-α and biological modifiers on cytokine production after astrocyte exposure to bilirubin: relationship to Nuclear Factor-kB. *Pediatr. Res., 55, [4, Part 2]*, 473A.

Fernandes, A.; Silva, R. F.; Falcão, A. S.; Brito, M. A. & Brites, D. (2004b). Cytokine production, glutamate release and cell death in rat cultured astrocytes treated with unconjugated bilirubin and LPS. *J Neuroimmunol, 153*, 64-75.

Genc, S.; Genc, K.; Kumral, A.; Baskin, H. & Ozkan, H. (2003). Bilirubin is cytotoxic to rat oligodendrocytes in vitro. *Brain Res, 985*, 135-141.

Gourley, G. R. (1997). Bilirubin metabolism and kernicterus. *Adv Pediatr, 44*, 173-229.

Green, D. R. & Reed, J. C. (1998). Mitochondria and apoptosis. *Science, 281*, 1309-1312.

Greenwalt, T. J. & Dumaswala, U. J. (1988). Effect of red cell age on vesiculation in vitro. *Br J Haematol, 68*, 465-467.

Haga, Y.; Tempero, M. A. & Zetterman, R. K. (1996). Unconjugated bilirubin inhibits in vitro cytotoxic T lymphocyte activity of human lymphocytes. *Biochim Biophys Acta, 1317*, 65-70.

Hankø, E.; Hansen, T. W. R.; Almaas, R.; Lindstad, J. & Rootwelt, T. (2005). Bilirubin induces apoptosis and necrosis in human NT2-N neurons. *Pediatr Res, 57*, 179-184.

Hansen, T. W. R. (2002). Mechanisms of bilirubin toxicity: clinical implications. *Clin Perinatol, 29*, 765-778.

Hansen, T. W. R. (2000). Kernicterus in term and near-term infants - the specter walks again. *Acta Paediatr, 89*, 1155-1157.

Hansen, T. W. R.; Maynard, E. C.; Cashore, W. & Oh, W. (1993). Endotoxemia and brain bilirubin in the rat. *Biol Neonate, 63*, 171-176.

Kaplan, M. & Hammerman, C. (2004). Understanding and preventing severe neonatal hyperbilirubinemia: is bilirubin neurotoxity really a concern in the developed world? *Clin Perinatol, 31*, 555-575.

Karp, W. B. (1979). Biochemical alterations in neonatal hyperbilirubinemia and bilirubin encephalopathy: a review. *Pediatrics, 64*, 361-368.

Kaufmann, N. A.; Simcha, A. J. & Blondheim, S. H. (1967). The uptake of bilirubin by blood cells from plasma and its relationship to the criteria for exchange transfusion. *Clin Sci, 33*, 201-208.

Keshavan, P.; Schwemberger, S. J.; Smith, D. L.; Babcock, G. F. & Zucker, S. D. (2004). Unconjugated bilirubin induces apoptosis in colon cancer cells by triggering mitochondrial depolarization. *Int J Cancer, 112*, 433-445.

Kroemer, G.; Dellaporta, B. & Resche-Rigon, M. (1998). The mitochondrial death/life regulator in apoptosis and necrosis. *Annu Rev Physiol, 60*, 619-642.

Kumral, A.; Genc, S.; Genc, K.; Duman, N.; Tatli, M.; Sakizli, M. & Ozkan, H. (2005). Hyperbilirubinemic serum is cytotoxic and induces apoptosis in murine astrocytes. *Biol Neonate, 87*, 99-104.

Lees, G. J. (1991). Inhibition of sodium-potassium-ATPase: a potentially ubiquitous mechanism contributing to central nervous system neuropathology. *Brain Res Brain Res Rev, 16*, 283-300.

Lin, S.; Yan, C.; Wei, X.; Paul, S. M. & Du, Y. (2003). p38 MAP kinase mediates bilirubin-induced neuronal death of cultured rat cerebellar granule neurons. *Neurosci Lett, 353*, 209-212.

Lindo, L.; Iborra, F. J.; Azorin, I.; Gueri, C. & Renau-Piqueras, J. (1993). Analysis of the endocytic-lysosomal system (vacuolar apparatus) in astrocytes during proliferation and differentiation in primary culture. *Int J Dev Biol, 37*, 565-572.

Liu, Y.; Peterson, D. A.; Kimura, H. & Schubert, D. (1997). Mechanism of cellular 3-(4,5-dimethylthiazol-2-yl)-2,5-diphenyltetrazolium bromide (MTT) reduction. *J Neurochem, 69*, 581-593.

Maisels, M. J. & Newman, T. B. (1995). Kernicterus in otherwise healthy, breast-fed term newborns. *Pediatrics, 96*, 730-733.

Maisels, M. J. & Newman, T. B. (1998). Jaundice in full-term and near-term babies who leave the hospital within 36 hours. The pediatrician's nemesis. *Clin Perinatol, 25*, 295-302.

Makar, T. K.; Nedergaard, M.; Preuss, A.; Gelbard, A. S.; Perumal, A. S. & Cooper, A. J. (1994). Vitamin E, ascorbate, glutathione, glutathione disulfide, and enzymes of glutathione metabolism in cultures of chick astrocytes and neurons: evidence that astrocytes play an important role in antioxidative processes in the brain. *J Neurochem, 62*, 45-53.

Malik, G. K.; Goel, G. K.; Vishwanathan, P. N.; Misra, P. K. & Sharma, B. (1986). Free and erythrocyte-bound bilirubin in neonatal jaundice. *Acta Paediatr Scand, 75*, 545-549.

Mayer, M. (2000). Association of serum bilirubin concentration with risk of coronary artery disease. *Clin Chem, 46*, 1723-1727.

Mayor, F. Jr.; Díez-Guerra, J.; Valdivieso, F. & Mayor, F. (1986). Effect of bilirubin on the membrane potential of rat brain synaptosomes. *J Neurochem, 47*, 363-369.

McDonagh, A. F. (1990). Is bilirubin good for you? *Clin Perinatol, 17*, 359-369.

McDonald, J. W.; Shapiro, S. M.; Silverstein, F. S. & Johnston, M. V. (1998). Role of glutamate receptor-mediated excitotoxicity in bilirubin-induced brain injury in the Gunn rat model. *Exp Neurol, 150*, 21-29.

Meldrum, B. S. (2000). Glutamate as a neurotransmitter in the brain: review of physiology and pathology. *J Nutr, 130*, 1007S-1015S.

Mireles, L. C.; Lum, M. A. & Dennery, P. A. (2000). Antioxidant and cytotoxic effects of bilirubin on neonatal erythrocytes. *Pediatr Res, 45*, 355-362.

Mollen, T. J.; Scarfone, R. & Harris, M. C. (2004). Acute, severe bilirubin encephalopathy in a newborn. *Pediatr Emerg Care, 20*, 599-601.

Moreau-Clevede, J. & Pays, M. (1979). Détermination de la bilirubine érythrocytaire. *Ann Biol Clin, 37*, 95-101.

Newman, T. B. & Maisels, M. J. (1992). Evaluation and treatment of jaundice in the term newborn: a kinder, gentler approach. *Pediatrics, 89*, 809-818.

Ngai, K. C. & Yeung, C. Y. (1999). Additive effect of tumor necrosis factor-α and endotoxin on bilirubin cytotoxicity. *Pediatr Res, 45*, 526-530.

Ngai, K. C.; Yeung, C. Y. & Leung, C. S. (2000). Difference in susceptibilities of different cell lines to bilirubin damage. *J Paediatr Child Health, 36*, 51-55.

Notter, M. F. & Kendig, J. W. (1986). Differential sensitivity of neural cells to bilirubin toxicity. *Exp Neurol, 94*, 670-682.

Ochoa, E. L. M.; Wennberg, R. P.; An, Y.; Tandon, T.; Takashima, T.; Nguyen, T. & Chui, A. (1993). Interactions of bilirubin with isolated presynaptic nerve terminals: functional effects on the uptake and release of neurotransmitters. *Cell Mol Neurobiol, 13*, 69-86.

Ostrow, J. D.; Mukerjee, P. & Tiribelli, C. (1994). Structure and binding of unconjugated bilirubin: relevance for physiological and pathophysiological function. *J Lip Res, 35*, 1715-1737.

Ostrow, J. D.; Pascolo, L.; Brites, D. & Tiribelli, C. (2004). Molecular basis of bilirubin-induced neurotoxicity. *Trends Mol Med, 10*, 65-70.

Ostrow, J. D.; Pascolo, L.; Shapiro, S. M. & Tiribelli, C. (2003). New concepts in bilirubin encephalopathy. *Eur J Clin Invest, 33*, 988-997.

Palmer, R. H.; Keren, R.; Maisels, M. J. & Yeargin-Allsopp, M. (2004). National Institute of Child Health and Human Development (NICHD) conference on kernicterus: a population perspective on prevention of kernicterus. *J Perinatol, 24*, 723-725.

Rashid, H.; Ali, M. K. & Tayyab, S. (2000). Effect of pH and temperature on the binding of bilirubin to human erythrocyte membranes. *J Biosci, 25*, 157-161.

Reiser, D. J. (2004). Neonatal jaundice: physiologic variation or pathologic process. *Crit Care Nurs Clin North Am, 16*, 257-269.

Rettig, M. P.; Low, P. S.; Gimm, J. A.; Mohandas, N.; Wang, J. & Christian, J. A. (1999). Evaluation of biochemical changes during in vivo erythrocyte senescence in the dog. *Blood, 93*, 376-384.

Rhine, W. D.; Schmitter, S. P.; Yu, A. C.; Eng, L. F. & Stevenson, D. K. (1999). Bilirubin toxicity and differentiation of cultured astrocytes. *J Perinatol, 19*, 206-211.

Rodrigues, C. M. P.; Solá, S.; Castro, R. E.; Laires, P. A.; Brites, D. & Moura, J. J. G. (2002a). Perturbation of membrane dynamics in nerve cells as an early event during bilirubin-induced apoptosis. *J Lipid Res, 43*, 885-894.

Rodrigues, C. M. P.; Solá, S. & Brites, D. (2002b). Bilirubin induces apoptosis via the mitochondrial pathway in developing rat brain neurons. *Hepatology, 35*, 1186-1195.

Rodrigues, C. M. P.; Solá, S.; Brito, A.; Brites, D. & Moura, J. J. G. (2002c). Bilirubin directly disrupts membrane lipid polarity and fluidity, protein order, and redox status in rat mitochondria. *J Hepatol, 36*, 335-341.

Rodrigues, C. M. P.; Solá, S.; Silva, R. & Brites, D. (2000). Bilirubin and amyloid-β peptide induce cytochrome *c* release through mitochondrial membrane permeabilization. *Mol Med, 6*, 936-946.

Rodrigues, C. M. P.; Solá, S.; Silva, R. F. M. & Brites, D. (2002d). Aging confers different sensitivity to the neurotoxic properties of unconjugated bilirubin. *Pediatr Res, 51*, 112-118.

Roseth, S.; Hansen, T. W. R.; Fonnum, F. & Walaas, S. I. (1998). Bilirubin inhibits transport of neurotransmitters in synaptic vesicles. *Pediatr Res, 44*, 312-316.

Savolainen, K. M.; Tervo, P.; Loikkanen, J. & Naarala, J. (1996). Cholinergic and glutaminergic excitation of neuronal cells. *ATLA, 24*, 387-392.

Schiff, D.; Chan, G. & Poznansky, M. J. (1985). Bilirubin toxicity in neural cell lines N115 and NBR10A. *Pediatr Res, 19*, 908-911.

Schinder, A. F.; Olson, E. C.; Spitzer, N. C. & Montal, M. (1996). Mitochondrial dysfunction is a primary event in glutamate neurotoxicity. *J Neurosci, 16*, 6125-6133.

Schmuck, G.; Röhrdanz, E.; Tran-Thi, Q. H.; Kahl, R. & Schlüter, G. (2002). Oxidative stress in rat cortical neurons and astrocytes induced by paraquat in vitro. *Neurotox Res, 4*, 1-13.

Seubert, J. M.; Darmon, A. J.; El Kadi, A. O.; D'Souza, S. J. & Bend, J. R. (2002). Apoptosis in murine hepatoma hepa 1c1c7 wild-type, C12, and C4 cells mediated by bilirubin. *Mol Pharmacol, 62*, 257-264.

Sharma, R. & Premachandra, B. R. (1991). Membrane-bound hemoglobin as a marker of oxidative injury in adult and neonatal red blood cells. *Biochem Med Metab Biol, 46*, 33-44.

Silva, R.; Mata, L. R.; Gulbenkian, S.; Brito, M. A.; Tiribelli, C. & Brites, D. (1999). Inhibition of glutamate uptake by unconjugated bilirubin in cultured cortical rat astrocytes: role of concentration and pH. *Biochem Biophys Res Commun, 265*, 67-72.

Silva, R. F. M., Falcão, A. S., Fernandes, A., Brito, M. A. & Brites, D. (2004). Is the bilirubin-induced release of glutamate from astrocytes calcium-dependent? *4th Forum of European Neuroscience*, 273A.

Silva, R. F. M.; Mata, L. R.; Gulbenkian, S. & Brites, D. (2001a). Endocytosis in rat cultured astrocytes is inhibited by unconjugated bilirubin. *Neurochem Res, 26*, 791-798.

Silva, R. F. M.; Rodrigues, C. M. P. & Brites, D. (2001b). Bilirubin-induced apoptosis in cultured rat neural cells is aggravated by chenodeoxycholic acid but prevented by ursodeoxycholic acid. *J Hepatol, 34*, 402-408.

Silva, R. F. M.; Rodrigues, C. M. P. & Brites, D. (2002). Rat cultured neuronal and glial cells respond differently to toxicity of unconjugated bilirubin. *Pediatr Res, 51*, 535-541.

Stocker, R.; Yamamoto, Y.; McDonagh, A. F.; Glazer, A. N. & Ames, B. N. (1987). Bilirubin is an antioxidant of possible physiological importance. *Science, 235*, 1043-1046.

Stout, A. K.; Raphael, H. M.; Kanterewicz, B. I.; Klann, E. & Reynolds, I. J. (1998). Glutamate-induced neuron death requires mitochondrial calcium uptake. *Nat Neurosci, 1*, 366-373.

Tsakiris, S. (1993). Na$^+$,K$^{(+)}$-ATPase and acetylcholinesterase activities: changes in postnatally developing rat brain induced by bilirubin. *Pharmacol Biochem Behav, 45*, 363-368.

Vázquez, J.; García-Calvo, M.; Valdivieso, F.; Mayor, F. & Mayor, F. Jr. (1988). Interaction of bilirubin with the synaptosomal plasma membrane. *J Biol Chem, 263*, 1255-1265.

Vetvicka, V.; Síma, P.; Miler, I. & Bilej, M. (1991). The immunosuppressive effects of bilirubin. *Folia Microbiol, 36*, 112-119.

Vítek, L.; Kotal, P.; Jirsa, M.; Malina, J.; Èerná, M.; Chmelar, D. & Fevery, J. (2000). Intestinal colonization leading to fecal urobilinoid excretion may play a role in the pathogenesis of neonatal jaundice. *J Pediatr Gastroenterol Nutr, 30*, 294-298.

Watchko, J. F. & Maisels, M. J. (2003). Jaundice in low birthweight infants: pathobiology and outcome. *Arch Dis Child Fetal Neonatal Ed, 88*, F455-F458.

Whittaker, V. P. (1993). Thirty years of synaptosome research. *J Neurocytol, 22*, 735-742.

Yamada, N.; Sawasaki, Y. & Nakajima, H. (1977). Impairment of DNA synthesis in Gunn rat cerebellum. *Brain Res, 126*, 295-307.

Yeung, C. Y. & Ngai, K. C. (2001). Cytokine- and endotoxin-enhanced bilirubin cytotoxicity. *J Perinatol, 21 Suppl 1*, S56-S58.

Zakim, D. & Wong, P. T. T. (1990). A high-pressure, infrared spectroscopic study of the solvation of bilirubin in lipid bilayers. *Biochemistry, 29*, 2003-2007.

Zucker, S. D.; Horn, P. S. & Sherman, K. E. (2004). Serum bilirubin levels in the U.S. population: gender effect and inverse correlation with colorectal cancer. *Hepatology, 40*, 827-835.

Zucker, S. D.; Storch, J.; Zeidel, M. L. & Gollan, J. L. (1992). Mechanism of the spontaneous transfer of unconjugated bilirubin between small unilamelar phosphatidylcholine vesicles. *Biochemistry, 31*, 3184-3192.

In: New Trends in Brain Research
Editor: F. J. Chen, pp. 39-60

ISBN 1-59454-834-X
© 2006 Nova Science Publishers, Inc.

Chapter II

DNA ENDOREPLICATION:
WHAT YOU DID NOT EXPECT FROM NEURONS

*L. Mola[1], M. Mandrioli[*2], B. Cuoghi[1] and D. Sonetti[2]*

[1] Department of Paleobiology Museum and Botanical Garden, Anatomical Museums,
University of Modena and Reggio Emilia, Modena, Italy
[2] Department of Animal Biology, University of Modena and Reggio Emilia,
Modena, Modena, Italy

ABSTRACT

Endoreplication has been repeatedly found in eukaryotes. In particular, endoreplicative or endoduplicative mechanisms have been reported in protists, plants, arthropods, molluscs, fish and mammals. The same studies indicated that cells possessing endoreplicated genome are generally large-sized and highly metabolically active, suggesting that endoreplication could have a functional significance. Neurons are typically considered as fully differentiated, non-dividing cells containing normally a diploid DNA amount, and endoreplication has not been historically reported in neuronal cells. Despite this general rule, some papers questioned the validity of this finding and indicated that giant neurons in molluscs, supramedullary and hypothalamic magnocellular neurons in fish and Purkinje cells in vertebrate, prevalently mammal cerebellum present DNA contents greater than 2C. Quantitative microfluorometric evaluation of DNA content in nerve cells of the gastropod molluscs *Planorbarius corneus, Aplysia californica* and *Lymnaea stagnalis* indicated that neuronal DNA contents are scattered between 2C and 200.000C values. This increase in DNA content is given in account mostly to whole-genome duplications, whereas in *P. corneus* an endoreplication mainly of GC-rich sequences occurs. The second example of endoreplicated neurons was highlighted in the large clustered neurons, located at the boundary between the *medulla oblongata* and spinal cord, of the fishes *Lophius piscatorius* and *Diodon holacanthus*. The DNA content of these neurons, evaluated by microfluorimetric methods, results ranging from a minimum

---

[*] E-mail: mola.lucrezia@unimore.it

of 4C in the smaller to over 5000C in the larger neurons. Further experiments with AT and GC specific fluorochromes showed that the increase in DNA content is due to an amplification involving GC-rich DNAs in *L. piscatorius*, whereas a whole-genome endoduplication occurs in *D. holacanthus*. Subsequent quantitative evaluation revealed that also *L. piscatorius* hypothalamic magnocellular neurons, located in the preoptic and tuberal complexes, largely exceed 2C DNA content. The last example is represented by nuclei of vertebrate Purkinje cells isolated from cerebellum. These results have been debated for several years, since contrasting data are present in literature. Up till now, the dilemma remains unsolved, but it is not possible to exclude that a small percentage of Purkinje neurons contains hyperdiploid and tetraploid nuclei, might be due to an extra DNA synthesis. In order to go in depth in the understanding of this topic, in the present review we revised the available data about endoreplication in invertebrate and vertebrate giant neurons and considered the possible molecular mechanisms responsible for endoreplication. Furthermore, some possible functional significances of neuron endoploidy are discussed.

INTRODUCTION

The mechanisms involved in the control of cell cycle are generally highly conserved in eukaryotes. However, some species possess cell cycle variations and, consequently, different control mechanisms of cell cycle [45].

One of the most common cell cycle variant is represented by endoreplication, in which cells increase their genomic DNA content without dividing. In particular, endoreplication is responsible for the presence of genomic DNA extra copies. In many cases the chromosome number is increased in multiples of N (the normal haploid chromosome number) bringing to cells that are referred to as polyploid or endopolyploid. On the contrary, in some cases, such as in the dipteran insects *Drosophila melanogaster* and *Chironomus thummi*, endoreplicated sister chromatids remain closely associated bringing to polytene chromosomes [45]. The best-known example of polyteny is found in the giant salivary gland chromosomes of *D. melanogaster*, which have up to 2048 copies of the euchromatic genome neatly aligned in parallel arrays [e.g. 121].

Although endoreplication is a dismissed evolutionary peculiarity, endoduplicated genomes result widespread in protists, plants and animals (including arthropods, molluscs, and mammals). Endocycling cells can become largely polyploid with C values (C value indicates the DNA content as a multiple of the normal haploid genome size) as high as 24000C as reported in some plants [120]. Considering that cell size is generally proportional to the amount of nuclear DNA, endoreplication constitutes an effective strategy for cellular growth and it is often found in differentiated cells that are large-sized or highly metabolically active.

Endoreplication is widespread in arthropods and it has been extensively studied in *D. melanogaster* [124]. In particular, polyploidy is a pervasive phenomenon in *Drosophila* and it occurs in both somatic tissues and derivatives of the germ-line. Examples include the nurse cells and follicle cells of the egg chamber within the female ovary. Genome-wide endoreplication is observed in both the nurse cells and follicle cells and during this process endoreplication mimics a normal cell cycle that alternates S phases and G phases, but without any M phase [45]. Following the cell-proliferative phase of *Drosophila* embryogenesis, many tissues initiate endocycles that lack all visible aspects of mitosis [112]. These tissues, which include gut, epidermis, fat body, malpighian tubules, trachea and salivary glands, continue to endocycle during larval development long after they are fully differentiated. Some adult tissues, including ovarian follicle and nurse cells and the sensory neurons in the wing, also employ endocycles. Final DNA levels in the larval cells appear to be developmentally programmed ranging from 16C to 2048C depending on cell type [45].

Endoreplication cycles were also reported in other insects and in particular in the nuclei of ovarian nurse and follicle cells of the silk moth *Hyalophora cecropia* [32] and in the salivary glands of the dipteran *Sciara coprophila* [74]. A unique feature of *S. coprophila* salivary gland polytene chromosomes is that certain loci form large "DNA puffs" in late larval life, which are sites not only of intense transcription but also of DNA amplification [56].

Cell types that undergo endoreplication were identified also in vertebrates and in particular in mammals [45]. An example is represent by megakaryocytes (blood cell type specialized to produce platelets) that, as a part of their differentiation process, become polyploid up to 128C [125]. Endopolyploidy is achieved via endomitosis and it is triggered by the secreted signal thrombopoietin. The large increase in megakaryocyte size that results from polyploidy is correlated with their ability to bud off adequate numbers of platelets. Endomitosis in megakaryocytes involves nuclear envelope breakdown and the appearance of condensed chromosomes and multipolar spindles [95]. Sister chromatids have been observed to separate in anaphase, but anaphase does not occur. As a consequence, replicated copies of chromosomes are incorporated into the same nucleus when the nuclear envelope reforms at a stage equivalent to telophase. Cytokinesis appears to be completely suppressed.

A second mammalian cell type that undergoes endocycles is represented by trophoblasts, which contribute to the placenta, that increase their DNA content to more than 1000C, presumably to face the high metabolic activity required to them [123, 129]. The chromosomes of trophoblast giant cells have regions in which replicated copies are tightly associated [123]. Thus their chromosomes are polytene, although they are not aligned along their entire lengths to produce the intricate banding patterns seen in insect polytene chromosomes.

Endoreplication has not been historically reported in neuronal cells that are typically considered as fully differentiated, non-dividing cells containing normally a diploid amount of DNA. Despite this general rule, some papers questioned the validity of this finding and indicated that giant neurons in molluscs, supramedullary and hypothalamic magnocellular neurons in fishes and Purkinje cells in vertebrate (prevalently mammals) cerebellum present DNA contents greater than 2C. In order to go in depth in the understanding of this topic, we revised in the present review the available data about endoreplication in invertebrate and vertebrate large sized neurons. Furthermore, some possible functional significances about neuron endoploidy are discussed.

SWITCHING FROM MITOSIS TO ENDOREPLICATION CYCLES

The endopolyploid state occurs when cells do not stop cycling when they become post-mitotic, but switch to an endoreplication cycle in which repeated S phases occur without intervening mitoses [44, 45].

Up to date, there are no papers that deal about the molecular mechanisms involved in neuron endoreplication. On the contrary endoreplication has been dissected at a molecular level in *Drosophila* evidencing several features that could fit neuron biology.

In *Drosophila*, the switch to endoreplication appears to be accomplished by loss of the mitotic cyclins A and B, while periodic expression of the S phase-promoter cyclin E continues [109]. Similar observations have been made in endoreplicating maize endosperm and in several mutants in yeast [110]. The increase in cdk activity that triggers DNA replication in yeast also makes replication origin complexes incapable of re-initiation [43]. This block to re-initiation is preserved during late S and G2 by the accumulation of the mitosis-promoting cyclin-cdks and removed when these complexes are inactivated by cyclin degradation at mitosis [43, 44, 110]. Thus, the absence of mitotic cyclins in endoreplicating cells may explain both the lack of mitosis and why re-initiation is no longer dependent on mitosis, whereas periodic cyclin E expression provides an explanation for how multiple rounds of DNA replication are triggered. Consistent with these ideas, inactivation of cdk1 complexes in *Drosophila* does not just arrest cells in G2, but forces them into an endoreplication cycle [44]. Moreover, although the pulses of cyclin E expression that normally precede each S phase during endoreduplication are necessary and sufficient to trigger S phases, periodic endoreplication can be inhibited by simply over-expressing cyclin E continuously.

A second set of molecules that resulted involved in endocycle switch on is represented by the Myc/Max/Mad network of transcription factors that plays a role in a wide range of cellular processes including growth and proliferation, differentiation, apoptosis and oncogenesis [58]. Members of the Myc family are found over-expressed in a wide variety of human tumors and are implicated in tumor initiation and progression. When ectopically expressed in mammalian cells, Myc proteins can induce proliferation and growth, block terminal differentiation and, in cooperation with other signals, induce transformation [58]. Conversely, over-expression of Mad family members leads to the arrest of the cell cycle in G1 [126].

The Myc/Max/Mad network is conserved in *Drosophila* and comprises dMax and single members of the Myc and Mad families, dMyc and dMnt, respectively [54, 104]. In particular, dMyc over-expression is present in endoreplicating cells resulting in dramatic increases in nuclear DNA content and cell and nucleolar size, whereas dMnt overexpression has the opposite effect. Ectopic expression of dMyc results in increased cytoplasmic and nuclear volume, as well as in enlarged nucleoli, as detected by increased anti-fibrillarin staining [104]. Fibrillarin has been implicated as a Myc target gene in both vertebrate and *Drosophila* cells [98, 104] and its increased expression is consistent with the notion that dMyc/Myc promotes ribosome biogenesis [104, 119]. dMyc can post-transcriptionally increase cyclin E levels in wing discs and studies in mammalian cells suggest that Myc can indirectly induce cyclin E expression [104]. Microarray analysis did not identify cyclin E as a transcriptional target of dMyc [104], suggesting that the transcriptional oscillation of cyclin E is not directly regulated by dMyc. Thus, dMyc is unable to drive endoreplication in the absence of normal cdk activity. Although the level of fibrillarin staining was not quantified, dMyc appears to drive somewhat more nucleolar growth than DNA accumulation when co-expressed with cyclin E or p21, indicating that dMyc may be able to drive a limited amount of nucleolar growth in the absence of DNA replication [104].

Experiments of BrdU staining of *Drosophila* follicle cells showed that endoreplication is not at whole-genome level since only four regions undergo localized amplification: two of these regions, or "amplicons," are located on the X chromosome and on chromosome 3 [22,

31]. In both cases, amplification is controlled by defined *cis*-acting elements that control the selective increase in chorion gene copy number [2, 4]. Both amplicons have been extensively characterized during the past 20 years and there are several evidences suggesting that the increase in chorion gene copy number is essential for the production of the large quantities of the encoded proteins required for the structural integrity of the eggshell [2, 4]. Linked genes within the amplicons are thought to "go along for the ride" by virtue of their proximity to the chorion genes. The amplification program is exquisitely controlled and is dependent upon the repression of replication at chromosomal positions except for those regions encompassing the amplicon [2, 4, 22]. Amplicons might exhibit variable levels of replication in different follicle cells. For example, at late stages of maturation the anterior-dorsal follicle cells seem to incorporate more BrdU than other follicle cells of the egg chamber, indicating that there is both a spatial and temporal control in the replication process [22].

A closer glance at *Drosophila* endocycles indicated that some genomic compartments are generally not endoreplicated. For example, in most polytene tissues centromeric and intercalary heterochromatin and telomeric sequences, that as a whole constitute approximately 30% of the *Drosophila* genome, are under-replicated. In addition, certain euchromatic regions, such as the histone genes, can be under-replicated [59, 68].

These data, as a whole, are very interesting since they can explain the occurrence of endoreplication also in neurons. In particular it could be possible to endoreplicate different genomic portions that contain genes whose expression is essential for the production of large quantities of proteins required for cell structural integrity and functioning. This hypothesis is strengthened by data indicating that endoreplicating cells are generally highly metabolically active. Finally, the mechanisms reported in *Drosophila* indicate that endoreplication occurs in the absence of mitosis and this is an essential element for neurons that are normally thought as non-diving cells and for this reason have specific mitotic blocking mechanisms.

GIANT NEURONS IN GASTROPOD MOLLUSKS

The nervous system of invertebrates represents an intriguing and important evolutionary step for neurobiological studies. Actually, invertebrates show very diversified organizations that range from the first nervous system appeared in Celentherata, in form of a spread network of few hundreds of small neurons, to the most complex invertebrate central nervous system (CNS) found in the cephalopod mollusc *Octopus* that reaches a relatively sophisticated organization comparable at least to that of the lower vertebrates, which behaviorally shows a relative high degree of "intelligence" and learning capabilities.

Giant nerve cells were found in a variety of invertebrates but, apart the special case of gastropod molluscs, where this peculiarity is almost the rule, they are not very frequent. Anyway, large and giant cells are only a component of these nervous systems, having the majority of the neurons small dimensions.

The first reported cases of giant nerve cells concern with nematode and annelids worms [for a review see reference n. 30] and in particular invertebrate neurophyisiologists studied extensively the giant Retzius cells, a couple of very large neurons located in segmental ganglia of the leech *Hirudo medicinalis*, that probably represent the first biochemically characterized neurons [37, 55]. Even in arthropods large neurons are present: Diptera,

Odonata, Chelicerata and Aracnoidea are reported to possess some giant elements [30]. These neurons, identified as motor elements, usually have large sized axonal fibers innervating major motor units and are responsible for rapid movements in response to visual stimuli as a reflex component to promote escape or aggressive behavior (the impulse transmission speed in unmielinated fiber is directly proportional to the axon diameter). At our knowledge, no reports concerns with the amount of DNA in the nuclei of these neurons.

In the different classes of molluscs, starting from the most primitive ones, we can assist to an increasing number of neurons and consequent complexity of CNS organization from a "cord-like" CNS to the advent of the ganglionic organization and "cephalization" of the CNS in form of aggregates of nerve cells in special well defined districts, the ganglia, gathered by nervous connectives and commissures in a ring encircling the oesophageal tube in proximity to the buccal complex. Each ganglion has a name justifying his innervation area and consequent function, i.e. buccal, cerebral, pedal, visceral etc.

As concerns the ganglion cells of gastropods, Bullock and Horridge [30] described them as "extraordinary in providing the basis of a disproportionate fraction of our knowledge of neuronal cytology, because of the large size and accessibility of some of them..." and more "the largest cells are veritable giants, not only relative to others in the same animals but to the nerve cells in any group of animals and indeed to active cells in general, attaining diameters of 0.8 mm". Finally, the authors stated "They (the large and giant neurons) are especially notable for the size of the nucleus, which is commonly about two-thirds of the diameter of the cell."

In works specifically dealing with the morphology of the neuronal nuclei in Gastropods [36, 60, 105], the chromatin is described as being made by clumps of heterochromatin uniformly dispersed in a less deeply stained nucleoplasm. In *Planorbarius corneus*, the increase of nuclear volume is associated with both the increase of nucleoli number and the amount of perinucleolar chromatin [75].

On the trail of this first indications, Kandel and his group [46], in adopting for their research the sea-hare *Aplysia californica* (a marine opistobranch that successively becomes famous for fundamental studies on the cellular and molecular basis of behavior) made an early identification of almost all the very large cells (about 30 neurons) and some prominent cell clusters located in the abdominal ganglion. They made a morpho-functional mapping of the giant neurons and gave them an initial description: the largest neurons found are L10 and R2 reported to reach in adults a soma diameter of almost 1 mm and contain an ellipsoid nucleus with a long axis up to 500 μm in size, thus visible *in vivo* beneath the semitransparent connective sheath, even at naked eye! These large identifiable cells are already present in the ganglia of small juvenile and do not change in number whilst the number of the small cells increases during animal life. What causes the increase of the size of the largest neurons and instead the number of the smaller cells is not known yet. Probably depending by an intrinsic genetic program, but it is suggested it could be a response to an increased functional demands, i.e. a major need in innervating growing body areas to serve, depending of the specific functional role. Usually, small neurons are thought to be sensory cells whilst large neurons are motoneurons or interneurons with a role as central pattern generators [122]. As Kandel [64] states, "some (neuronal) cell types, often large cells may never vary in number because they never experience demands for functional elaboration, or if they do they respond enlarging and undergoing DNA replication but not cellular replication".

The neuronal large size and the possibility to identify and map the cells in specific location within the ganglia of several gastropod species, i.e. to find the corresponding individual cell in different specimens and sometimes even among different species, offered in the recent past to the investigators of different neuroresearch branches some practical advantages: single neurons were intracellularly recorded by electrophysiologists that wanted to identify type of activity and function in order to rebuilt neuronal circuity underlying specific behavioral responses whilst biochemists had the opportunity to study the chemical content of single cells in term of neurotransmitters and other neuromolecules of interest in a dynamic contest [for a review see reference n. 100]. The possibility to manipulate and isolate giant neurons with relative easy permitted to culture them *in vitro* in order to study under controlled parameters phenomena like neuro-degeneration/-regeneration in presence of microglial cells [113] or to rebuild *in vitro* simple neuronal networks or circuity [93]. Among the most mentioned giant neurons, in addition to those above reported in *A. californica*, there are the metacerebral serotonergic neurons of *Helix* [99], and the giant dopaminergic neuron in the pedal ganglion of *P. corneus* and *Lymnaea stagnalis* [1, 102]. The giant neurons are found in small but constant numbers in all the central ganglia at least in a variety of pulmonates and opisthobranchs, but seemingly not in prosobranchs so far examined; fewest occur in the buccal, pleural, and cerebral ganglia, most in the visceral and pedal ones.

The study of the DNA content of giant molluscan neurons was firstly faced by Coggeshall et al. [38]. Cytophotometric analyses have shown that the DNA content in giant neurons of *A. californica* can vary, during growth, from 2000C to 75000C by incremental duplications of the whole genome, thus supporting the occurrence of the phenomenon of poliploidy. The absence of selective duplication has been confirmed by fluorometric analyses, which have permitted the detection of giant neurons containing an amount of DNA 200000 times higher than the haploid 1 C value, found in spermatozoa of the same species [71]. Furthermore, a quantitative analysis of large nuclei after Feulgen DNA reactions revealed the presence of repeated duplication of whole genome in other gastropods, the pulmonates snails *Helix pomatia* [78] and *L. stagnalis* [19]. The DNA content in ganglion cells of molluscs, far in excess of both the 2C and 4C normal diploid values, has been the object of a number of successive studies [for review see reference n. 26].

Results in contrast with the previous ones were obtained in the freshwater snail *P. corneus* and the land snail *Achatina fulica* that indicate a differential duplication of DNA, rather than a repeated whole-genome duplication [34, 76, 77, 79]. Cytochemical and microfluorometric analyses, useful in discriminating GC-rich from AT-rich DNAs, suggested that during the development of the central nervous system in *P. corneus*, the increasing DNA content and consequent nuclear volume is due to a differential amplification of guanine-cytosine rich DNA sequences in selected compartments of the genome. These data indicate that the dispersion of DNA values is almost exclusively due to the extremely variable amounts of DNA and not to partially double stranded RNAs. Moreover, the results obtained by photo-oxidation of nuclei of different dimensions further shows that this technique is much more destructive when applied to DNA contained in giant and large nuclei. As noted by Chase and Tolloczko [34], differential DNA endoreplication of some DNA sequences or selective gene amplification is highest during the period of animal's greatest growth and then decline rapidly near the onset of sexual maturity.

Two mechanisms have been postulated to explain gene amplification: unequal mitotic crossing-over and disproportionate or saltatory replication of single tracts of DNA [67, 101]. Manicardi et al. [79] suggested that the model involving unequal crossing over seems unlikely, since the studied material was represented by nerve cells with suppressed mitotic phase. Instead, gene amplification in *P. corneus* is much more likely explained by the hypothesis of a saltatory replication of DNA, since, in this case, the appearance of additional rounds of replication produces a variable copy of amplified sequences [67, 101]. This model, already widely utilized to sustain several cases of gene amplification [106], can perhaps better explain the findings in *P. corneus* because it does not require the breakage of the original gene and furthermore, it is disengaged from the mitotic phase. Some other theoretical considerations can be made as to the reasons for gene amplification in mollusks. DNA amplification might concern genes involved in the synthesis of a specific neuropeptide: where there is a need for rapid synthesis of special gene products, it may inferred that the parts of the genome involved in such processes are the same as those that will be differentially replicated. Alternatively, the amplified genes might be involved in a more aspecific mechanism, as, for instance, the production of a considerable amount of rDNA aimed to generally increase protein synthesis capacity. In *A. californica* the investigations by Picciotto et al. [103] seem to exclude an amplification concerning genes codifying for neuropeptides. The same conclusion was reached in *L. stagnalis* by Smit (personal communication). Utilizing specific cDNA probes, this Author demonstrated by DNA hybridization experiments, that the massive production of a specific neurohormone is not related to an amplification of the corresponding structural gene. Therefore, the most plausible explanation of the data found in *P. corneus* is that the genomic amplified portions contain cistrons for the production of ribosomal RNA. Moreover this hypothesis is sustained by the particular abundance of GC sequences in the rDNA of many eukaryotes [111].

These data, as a whole, allow us to suggest that DNA over-replication could make a single neuronal large cell able to function as a substitute for a multiple cell system: in other words a giant molluscan neuron could be regarded as a "single cell ganglion" combining the properties of many equivalent cells. As it has been suggested, a giant neuron may assume more than one function i.e., it may include a motoneuron and interneuron or a sensory neuron and interneuron components. These multiple roles of large invertebrate neurons is also supported by the evidence that they produce more than one neurotransmitters. Immunohistochemical studies have shown the coexistence of two or more neuropeptides in the same elements that are produced by expression of different genes or by a differential cleavage of a common proteic precursor [114]. Recently Sonetti et al. [115] surmise that a neuronal population in *P. corneus* including large elements immunopositive both to anti-morphine and anti-ACTH antibodies constitutes a system devoted to trauma response: initially, they release ACTH-like material and thereafter, the same cells, by a "programmed" delay or by a feed-back signal system, release a morphine-like molecule to terminate or calming the state of alertness and cell activation and to re-establish the organism homeostasis, as first suggested by Stefano and Scharrer [117]. Comparing with other molluscan species, the Authors found that differences exist in expressing the coupling of these signaling families: in *Mytilus* as in humans large nerve cell bodies aren't present as in *P. corneus*, so *Mytilus* appears to have very similar association of these signaling families in different sets of cells, as found in man. On the contrary, *Planorbarius* solves this linkage problem having the link that takes place in the same large neurons as well as having it more spread out. Thus, the differences in the association all reveal that the coupling of these systems is always present but *Planorbarius*, as other gastropods solved the problem endowing the solution of different tasks carried on by the same large cell. A solution that showed evident adaptative limitations by the fact that very rarely the choice of giant neurons has been reproposed in vertebrates, as described in the following chapters.

SUPRAMEDULLARY NEURONS OF FISH

Large cells, named supramedullary neurons (SN), localized on the dorsal midline surface of spinal cord (under the external limiting membrane), are present in adult teleosts belonging to various orders. Credit should be given to Fritsch [47] for the discovery of these neurons in *Lophius*, then the studies on these peculiar nervous cells continued all the 20th century long and they are still intriguing and represent suitable models for molecular and *in vitro* investigations.

The SN are aligned along the spinal cord in a few orders (Clupeiformes, Syngnatiformes, Scorpaeniformes, Pleuronectiformes and Perciformes), while they are clustered at the rostral end in others (Tetraodontiformes, Lophiiformes and Batrachoidiformes). These neurons, have defined number and size for each species [for a complete review see reference n. 89]. Ultrastructural analysis showed that both aligned SN [85, 86, 90] and clustered SN [39, 40, 96] are engaged in a high synthetic activity with rapid turnover of cell structures. For example, the presence of abundant rough endoplasmic reticulum and well developped Golgi apparatus, together with the remarkably vesicular traffic in the cytoplasmic compartment, indicate an intense process of protein biosynthesis.

Studies on electrophysiological characteristics of SN demonstrated that these neurons, provided with an unmielinated axon, are efferent and coupled [10, 11, 12, 127] and morphological evidences about the existence of gap junctions were also demonstrated [13, 128]. These neurons show immunoreactivity to a gastrin/CCK-like peptide [5, 8, 53], ACTH-like peptide [42], noradrenaline [92] and nNOS [41]. Immunohistochemical, physiological and neuroanatomical data, taken together, pointed out that this neuronal system is a component of the autonomic nervous system [89]. The localization out of the spinal cord, the presence of noradrenaline [92] and the ending of the cells on mucous glands in the skin [53] are clear evidences of this statement. This neuronal system, through mucous secretion, may aid in protection from predation or may help in preventing infection from a wound that would follow a predatory strike [127].

Over the course of our investigations, it seemed that the nucleus of clustered SN in the angler fish *Lophius piscatorius* showed abundant chromatin than other neurons in the dorsal spinal cord. This prompted a number of research on the nucleus of these neurons.

Histochemical analysis on the nuclei of clustered SN in *L. piscatorius,* carried out using a computerized image analysis system, showed that the amount of DNA-Feulgen is higher than that in other spinal cord neurons [6].

DNA content of *L. piscatorius* SN was evaluated by microfluorimentric methods, using specimens ranging from 18-25 cm. Slides stained with ethidium bromide have given a DNA content ranging from 8C in the smaller neurons (nuclear diameter of 15 µm) to a maximum of 1158C in the larger ones (nuclear diameter of 60 µm), demonstrating a direct correlation between nuclear size and C value. The value obtained using Acriflavine Feulgen confirmed these findings [7]. Because the genome size for this species is 1 pg [33], these values correspond to a minimum of 8 pg and a maximum of 1158 pg. This result was the first exceptional finding for the nervous system of vertebrates.

The checking of larger specimens of L. *piscatorius* (about 30 cm) indicated that the DNA content of SN can reach more than 5000C, in relationship with both nuclear and animal size [108]. Utilization of AT and GC specific fluorochromes (DAPI and chromomycin A_3 respectively) showed that the increase in DNA content is due to differential genome amplification involving GC-rich DNA sequences. Indeed, as the nuclear size of the cluster neurons increases, GC-rich sequences increase more than AT-rich ones. These data suggested that over-replication of GC-rich sequences with respect to AT-rich sequences is also correlated with the increase in animal size. Nucleolar organizing region (NOR) staining, carried out with the aim of testing the involvement of the NORs in the increase of nuclear area, showed that each neuron of the cluster contains a single nucleolus [108]. Considering that both the DNA transcribing for specific mRNAs and the NORs transcribing for rRNAs, are generally rich in GC sequences, it has been suggested that the increase in GC-rich DNA found in the clustered SN is due to the need of increasing the transcriptional activity of some genes. An other hypothesis, which can justify the GC-rich sequences differential endoreplication, is that specific gene complexes are amplified for overproduction of peptides/proteins [108].

The DNA amplification is a general phenomenon for fish clustered SN, because recently cytofluorimetric research carried out in *Diodon holacanthus* (a teleost belonging to Tetraodontiformes, an order very distant from Lophiiformes) indicated a DNA content ranging from 4C (in the smaller nuclei with mean diameter of 30 µm) to more than 500C (in the larger nuclei with mean diameter of 60 µm) [91].

Ultrastructural studies performed on D. *holacanthus* SN nuclei revealed an unusually high chromatin content homogeneously dispersed in the karyoplasms, in agreement with the cytofluorimetric evaluation. Moreover, the nucleolar ultrastructural data, together with silver staining performed on D. *holacanthus* specimens, suggested an intense production of ribosomal components, which likely serve in order to satisfy high cellular demands for protein synthesis. Accordingly to this hypothesis, a remarkably high number of nuclear pores were observed, and this fits well with a high rate of nuclear metabolism and intense nuclear-cytoplasmic traffic [40].

In D. *holacanthus* SN nuclei the distribution of C values indicates an inter- and intra-individual variation in DNA content, which does not correspond to duplications of the whole genome, suggesting that DNA replication is differential for specific genes (endoreplication). Also in D. *holacanthus* the DNA content appears to be correlated with nuclear size, but the endoreplication occurs without preferential enrichment of either AT- or GC-rich DNA sequences [91]. Thus, the endoreplication pathways in this neuronal system are different from species to species.

Vertebrate neurons just rarely have a DNA content exceeding 2C so, on the whole, these research are surprising demonstrating, for the fist time, a DNA endoreplication in a specific neuronal type of vertebrates. The reliability of these results is based on the ease with which the SN of fish can be extracted and on their accurate identification, given their remarkable size and their typical localization.

HYPOTHALAMIC NEUROSECRETORY NEURONS OF FISH

The phenomenon of endoreplication was subsequently demonstrated in other large neurons of fish. Light microscopy analysis of histological sections treated with Feulgen reaction showed that the nucleus of the hypotalamic magnocellular neurons, located in the preoptic and tuberal complexes, are intensely stained in both *L. piscatorius* and *D. holacanthus* [9]. These findings were confirmed by computerized image analysis, measuring the total nuclear area, the integrated optic density (i.o.d.) and the i.o.d. per area unit. The analysis, carried out both on the hypothalamic neurosecretory neurons (preoptic and tuberal complexes) and on the surrounding glial and ependimal cells, showed that the i.o.d. per area unit is comparable in all the cells in question, indicating that the increase in the nuclear area of neurosecretory neurons is matched by an increase in their Feulgen-DNA content. The microfluorimetric analysis on slides treated with EB staining demonstrated that the hypotalamic neurons have nuclei whose DNA content increase with the increase of their size, reaching values of about 68C in *L. piscatorius* and about 84C in *D. holacanthus*. The relationship between the increase in nuclear area and that in DNA content follows a similar pattern in both species. The percent distributions of C values in the nuclei of hypothalamic neurons from these species show that, in general, the peaks did not correspond to integral multiples of the 2C diploid amount. This finding suggested that the increase in DNA amount might be due to differential genome amplification [9].

The data on hypothalamic neurosecretory neurons indicate that, in *L. piscatorius* and *D. holacanthus*, a marked increase of DNA content is not an exclusive feature of the supramedullary neuron cluster. It is possible a parallelism between the two cell types of fish. Hypothalamic neurosecretory neurons and SN share a large size and an intense biosynthetic activity (hormones and neuromediators respectively).

PURKINJE CELLS OF VERTEBRATE CEREBELLUM

The last example of endoreplication in vertebrate neurons is represented by nuclei of Purkinje cells isolated from cerebellum and other CNS cells, such as hippocampal pyramidal neurons. These results were a matter of controversy for almost thirty years (from about 1965 till the first years of nineties). Indeed, a DNA content higher than 2C is reported in a number of works [14, 16, 17, 18, 20, 21, 23, 24, 25, 27, 28, 29, 57, 62, 63, 66, 69, 70, 73, 80, 83, 97, 107, 118] whilst other Authors pointed out a DNA amount for these cells corresponding to normal 2C [35, 48, 49, 51, 52, 81, 82, 84, 88, 94].

Purkinje cells of the cerebellum were particularly often studied, like supramedullary neurons, because of their distinct morphology and easy and reliable identification. Many studies suggested that Purkinje cells DNA content exceed 2C and may amount to tetraploid or even octoploid levels in several mammals, such as human [69, 70, 80], cat [61, 62] and rat

[21, 73, 97, 107]. Other studies questioned the validity of these findings and assessed that Purkinje cell nuclei have diploid DNA content in rat [51, 81, 94], mouse [35, 81], rabbit and Guinea pig [81] and human [82, 84]. Differences in technical approach and measurement errors could be responsible for these conflicting data [52, 83]. Some Authors cleared that just the identification criteria of Purkinje cells, that are large volume of the nucleus, together with dense cytoplasm, can introduce artefacts in cytophotometry [50]. For these reasons, the importance of making appropriate corrections considering non specific factors for reliable measurements of DNA content was stressed [81].

In spite of these criticisms, a cytophotometric study of DNA content performed in Purkinje cells of rats, cats, chicken and humans revealed that in a certain number of cells the amount of DNA ranges between the diploid and tetraploid level. The incidence of tetraploid Purkinje cells vary among the species studied and great interindividual differences were observed. In rats, for instance, the incidence of these cells varies from 1 to 23 %. Densitometric analysis of the distribution of nuclear chromatin showed that tetraploid Purkinje cells are richer in condensed chromatin, especially in the region of the nucleolus, which apparently contains the surplus of DNA. It is proposed that the phenomenon of DNA hyperdiploidy arises as a result of either incomplete S-phase in some immature Purkinje cell precursors or the amplification of some DNA sequences particularly those localized in the nucleolar region [27].

A critical analysis of various cytophotometric, radioautographic and biochemical approaches to the problem of CNS neuron polyploidization revealed potentially serious flaws in many of them, rendering virtually impossible interpretation of the numerous contradictory results in the literature [118].

Although cytofluorimetric methods encompass an intrinsic error of about 10-15%, which may interfere with evaluations of small differences in DNA content, the existence of some "extra-DNA" (in the range 2.2C - 2.5C) in neuronal nuclei of human CNS (pre- and post-central girus, cerebellum cortex and spinal cord) was postulated [20]. The Authors suggested as possible interpretation that it may play an important role in the functional activity of the CNS.

Following studies about Purkinje neurons DNA-content in several vertebrate species such as rainbow trout, Amazon molly fish, salamander, mouse, rat, rabbit, cat, dog, monkey and human, showed a low incidence of Purkinje cell nuclei with interclass DNA amounts. Also a low frequency (1-7%) of Purkinje cell nuclei with 4C DNA levels was observed in all species examined, except salamander and rabbit [72, 87].

A relationship between the heterogeneity of Purkinje cell chromatin and the afferent systems of the cerebellum areas was suggested, comparing two stages of eel life cycle (yellow eel and silver eel) characterised by a different degree of swimming activity [16]. DNA content of Purkinje neurons was also related to hibernation in frog [3] and hedgehog [18]. These studies demonstrated that nuclear heterogeneity (diploid-hyperdiploid) in Purkinje cell population reflects differences in metabolic states. On the other hand, a link between the susceptibility of cells of the cerebellum to hypoxia and the amount of DNA also was more recently suggested [65].

Cerebellum of rat embryos was also transplanted into sensomotor cortex of adult rats and DNA content in granule and Purkinje cells of the transplant was determined cytophotometrically. Granule cells are diploid; about 3% Purkinje cells contain hyperdiploid and tetraploid nuclei, which correspond to the content of such cells in the adult cerebellum. Therefore, the data showed that cell hyperploidy does not depend on the functional load but is essential property of the tissue [87].

In the last years the discussion about Purkinje neurons faded a bit and, till now, the dilemma about polyploidy of Purkinje cells population remains unsolved. However, it is not possible to exclude that a small percentage of Purkinje neurons contains hyperdiploid and tetraploid nuclei, might be due to an extra DNA synthesis, the significance of which still remain to be cleared. In any case, this phenomenon may not be comparable with endoreplication in SN and hypothalamic neurosecretory neurons in which the DNA amount reaches such high values that are impossible to be confused or artefacted.

CONCLUSIONS

Given its widespread occurrence in evolutionary distant species and in highly different cell types, it is not easy to furnish an unique explanation about the role that endoduplication plays in cells. Nevertheless, at least two generalizations can be offered. In particular, a common element is that endoreplication is typical of large or metabolically active cells suggesting that endocycling is an effective tool to allow cells to increase their mass or metabolic output. Finally, since endoreplication permits growth without periodic rearrangements of cytoskeletal elements or cell-cell contacts, as happens in mitosis, it is less disruptive to highly structured tissues than is mitotic proliferation. Together these properties conspire to make endocycle an advantageous strategy for cells and tissues that even terminally differentiated yet must continue to grow.

These features are extremely interesting for neurons that are fully differentiated and non-dividing cells since they could improve their functional plasticity without disruptive effects on nervous system structure. The analysis of endoreplication phenomenon in neurons allows us to evidence some common elements that could explain endocycling occurrence in this peculiar cell type.

First of all, it should be stressed that giant or large-sized neurons even if found in a variety of invertebrate and vertebrate species, are generally not very frequent. In fact, if endoreplication presence is considered from an evolutionary perspective, it resulted as "reinvented" several times during evolution. In particular, the presence of a single polyploid cell may be considered as a substitute for the multiple cell system: in other words a giant or large neuron could be regarded as a "single cell ganglion" combining the properties of many equivalent cells. This evolutionary choice could be useful from a functional point of view since it allows the increase of cell functionality without affecting tissue structure or organization. However, the presence of a unique multifunctional and highly active neuron could represent an important weak point of the nervous system since makes it more susceptible to damage in respect to a multiple cell system that could be reorganized after a damage to a single cell. Moreover, a system made of several cells could be more efficient than a single large neuron in term of assuring a fine integration of the afferent signals and a successive elaboration of accurate responses to the received input.

A second common element among polyploid or endopolyploid neurons consists in the fact that neuron level of ploidy is directly related to animal size. This feature is not surprising since the increase in animal size could involve an increase in neuron functional requirements that can be faced though an enhancement of neuron ability in synthesizing peptides or other cellular components. This finding, therefore, reinforces our hypothesis that endocycling is an effective tool to increase cellular metabolic output.

DNA endoreplication can be obtained through rounds of amplification of specific gene sequences or by generalized whole-genome amplifications. At this regard, a discrepancy exists in the data reported in neurons since in the invertebrate species *A. californica, H. pomatia* and *L. stagnalis* the DNA content varies by incremental duplications of the whole genome, whereas in the land snail *A. fulica,* in the planorbid *P. corneus* and in all the described endoploid vertebrate neurons a differential duplication of specific DNA sequences rather than a repeated duplication of the whole genome is reported. This discrepancy could be due to the absence of clustering in amplicons of those genes whose amplification is necessary to satisfy neuron functional requirements in *A. californica, H. pomatia* and *L. stagnalis*. The presence of a DNA endoreplication consisting in rounds of amplification of specific gene instead of generalized whole-genome amplifications represents an evolutionary advantage since the amplification of unnecessary DNA sequences and/or "trash DNAs" can be avoided. Furthermore, the possibility to amplify different genes in each cell type will increase the functionality of endoreplication since it will be increased only those genes that are essential for the production of large quantities of proteins required for cell structural maintenance or functioning. Cells that play the same functions will therefore amplify mainly the same genes in view of the same functional needs.

A further apparent discrepancy consists in the presence of differences in the amplified genomic compartments since, for example *L. piscatorius* and *P. corneus* amplify predominantly GC-rich DNAs, whereas *D. holacanthus* and some molluscs did not showed any preferential AT or GC-rich DNA amplification. These results are only apparently controversial since amplicons can consist of genes whose proteins are essential for cells and DNA sequences that "go along for the ride" by virtue of their proximity to the functional important genes. This endoreplication feature suggests that the differential amplification that occurs for example in the fish *L. piscatorius* and *D. holacanthus* does not reflect different functions of SNs but only a difference in the type of genes that are amplified passively in virtue of their proximity to the functional important ones. This result could be simply due to difference in genome organization occurring in the two studied fish species that are phylogenetically distant. A similar hypothesis could also explain the data observed in mollusks.

Despite the amount of available results, a number of substantial and intriguing questions still remain. For example, what and why genetic programs mediate the switch from mitotic to endocycles? What programs define which cell types will undergo endoreplication? How frequently did novel mechanisms for endocycling arise during evolution, and how extreme are the variations in regulation? Answers to these questions promise to provide insights that pertain not only to endoreplication, but also to the mechanisms used in proliferative cycles and growth control.

REFERENCES

[1]   Audesirk, G. (1985). Amine-containing neurons in the brain of *Lymnaea stagnalis*: distribution and effects of precursors. *Comp. Biochem. Physiol. A., 81*, 359-65.

[2]   Austin, R. J., Orr-Weaver, T. L. & Bell, S. P. (1999). *Drosophila* ORC specifically binds to ACE3, an origin of DNA replication control element. *Genes Dev., 13*, 2639-2649.

[3]   Barni, S., Bernocchi, G. & Biggiogera, M. (1983). Chromatin organization in frog Purkinje neurons during the annual cycle: cytochemical and ultrastructural studies. *Bas. Appl. Histochem., 27*, 129-140.

[4]   Beall, E. L., Manak, J. R., Zhou, S., Bell, M., Lipsick, J. S. & Botchan, M. R. (2002). Role for a *Drosophila* Myb-containing protein complex in site-specific DNA replication. *Nature, 420*, 833–837.

[5]   Benedetti, I. & Mola, L. (1988). Survey of neuropeptide-like immunoreactivity in supramedullary neurons of *Coris julis* (L.). *Brain Res., 449*, 373-376.

[6]   Benedetti, I. & Mola, L. (1991). Preliminary findings on the nucleus of large neurons in *Lophius piscatorius* L. (Osteichthyes, Lophiiformes). *Eur. J. Appl. Histochem., 35*, 245-248.

[7]   Benedetti, I., Manicardi, G. C. & Mola, L. (1993). Cytofluorimetric determination of DNA content in large neurons of *Lophius piscatorius* L. (Osteichthyes, Lophiiformes). *Eur. J. Histochem., 37*, 91-95.

[8]   Benedetti, I., Mola, L., Marini, M. & Calzolari, C. (1993). Neuroanatomical and immunohistochemical studies on the dorsal neurons in the spinal cord of *Trigla lucerna* L. and *Scorpaena porcus* L. (Scorpaeniformes). *Ann. Anat., 175*, 77-80.

[9]   Benedetti, I., Sassi, D., Mescoli, G. & Manicardi, G. C. (1999). High values of DNA content in the hypotalamic neurons of *Lophius piscatorius* and *Diodon holacanthus* (Osteichthyes). *Caryologia, 52*, 141-146.

[10]   Bennett, M. L. V., Crain, S. M. & Grundfest, H. (1959). Electrophysiology of supramedullary neurons in *Sphaeroides maculatus*. I. Orthodromic and antidromic responses. *J. Gen. Physiol., 43*, 159-188.

[11]   Bennett, M. L. V., Crain, S. M. & Grundfest, H. (1959). Electrophysiology of supramedullary neurons in *Sphaeroides maculatus*. II. Properties of the electrically excitable membrane. *J. Gen. Physiol., 43*, 189-219.

[12]   Bennett, M. L. V., Crain, S. M. & Grundfest, H. (1959). Electrophysiology of supramedullary neurons in *Sphaeroides maculatus*. III. Organization of the supramedullary neurons. *J. Gen. Physiol., 43*, 221-250.

[13]   Bennett, M. L. V., Nakajima, Y. & Pappas, G. D. (1967). Physiology and ultrastructure of electrotonic junctions. I. Supramedullary neurons. *J. Neurophysiol., 30*, 161-179.

[14]   Bernocchi, G. (1983). Feulgen-DNA patterns of Purkinje cell population in vertebrates with different cerebellar cytoarchitectonics. *J. Hirnforsch., 24*, 35-42.

[15]   Bernocchi, G. (1985). Cytochemical variations in Purkinje neuron nuclei of cerebellar areas with different afferent systems in *Rana esculenta*. Comparison between activity and hibernation. *J. Hirnforsch, 26*, 659-665.

[16] Bernocchi, G. & Barni, S. (1985). On the heterogeneity of Purkinje neurons in vertebrates. Cytochemical and morphological studies of chromatin during eel (*Anguilla anguilla* L.) life cycle. *J. Hirnforsch., 26*, 227-235.

[17] Bernocchi, G. & Scherini, E. (1981). Maternal protein malnutrition and post-natal cerebellar histogenesis in the rat. Effects on feulgen-DNA content of Purkinje cell population. *Cell Mol. Biol. Incl. Cyto. Enzymol., 27*, 253-261.

[18] Bernocchi, G., Barni, S. & Scherini, E. (1986). The annual cycle of *Erinaceus europaeus* L. as a model for a further study of cytochemical heterogeneity in Purkinje neuron nuclei. *Neuroscience, 17*, 427-437.

[19] Boer, H. H., Groot, C., De Jong-Brink, M. & Cornelisse, C. J. (1977). Polyploidy in the freshwater snail *Lymnaea stagnalis* (Gastropoda Pulmonata), A cytophotometric analysis of the DNA in neurons and some other cell types. *Neth. J. Zool., 27*, 245-252.

[20] Bohm, N., Kroner, B. & Kaiser, E. (1981). Cytophotometric evidence of non-S-phase extra-DNA in human neuronal nuclei. *Cell Tissue Kinet., 14*, 433-444.

[21] Bohn, R. C. & Mitchell, R. B. (1976). Cytophotometric identification of tetraploid Purkinje cells in young and aged rats. *J. Neurobiol., 7*, 255-258.

[22] Botchan, M. & Levine, M. A. (2004). Genome analysis of endoreplication in the *Drosophila* ovary. *Dev. Cell, 6*, 4-5.

[23] Bregnard, A., Knusel, A. & Kuenzle, C. C. (1975). Are all the neuronal nuclei polyploid ? *Histochemistry, 43*, 59-62.

[24] Bregnard, A., Kuenzle, C. C. & Ruch, F. (1977). Cytophotometric and autoradiographic evidence for post-natal DNA synthesis in neurons of the rat cerebral cortex. *Exp. Cell Res., 107*, 151-157.

[25] Bregnard, A., Ruch, F., Lutz, H. & Kuenzle, C. C. (1979). Histones and DNA increase synchronously in neurons during early postnatal development of the rat forebrain cortex. *Histochemistry, 61*, 271-279.

[26] Brodsky, V. Y. & Uryvaeva, I. V. (1985). *Genome multiplication in growth and development,* Cambridge, UK: Cambridge University Press.

[27] Brodsky, V. Y., Marshak, T. L., Mares, V., Lodin, Z., Fulop, Z. & Lebedev, E. A. (1979). Constancy and variability in the content of DNA in cerebellar Purkinje cell nuclei. A cytophotometric study. *Histochemistry, 59*, 233-248.

[28] Brodsky, V. Y., Marshak, T. L., Mikeladze, Z. A., Moskovkin, G. N. & Sadykova, M. K. (1984). DNA synthesis in the Purkinje neurons. *Bas. Appl. Histochem., 28*, 187-194.

[29] Brodski, V. Y., Sokolova, G. A. & Manakova, T. E. (1971). Multiple increase of DNA in the Purkinje cells of cerebellum in ontogenesis of rats. *Ontogeny, 2*, 33-36.

[30] Bullock, T. H., & Horridge, G. A. (1965). *Structure and function in the nervous system of invertebrates.* vol. II. San Francisco, USA: Freeman & Co.

[31] Calvi, B. R., Lilly, M. A. & Spradling, A. C. (1998). Cell cycle control of chorion gene amplification. *Genes Dev., 12*, 734-744.

[32] Cardoen, J., Watson, C., Deloof, A., Spencer, A. & Berry J. (2005) Polyploidy in the nuclei of ovarian nurse and follicle cells of the silk moth, *Hyalophora cecropia. Arch. Insect Biochem. Physiol., 15*, 93- 100.

[33] Cavalier-Smith, T. (1991). Coevolution in vertebrate genome, cell and nuclear size. In G. Ghiara (Ed.), *Selected Symposia and monographs: Symposium of the evolution of terrestrial vertebrates* (pp. 51-86). Modena, Italy: Mucchi.

[34] Chase, R. & Tolloczko, B. (1987). Evidence for differential DNA endoreplication during the development of a molluscan brain. *J. Neurobiol., 18*, 395-406.

[35] Cohen, J., Mares, V. & Lodin, Z. (1973). DNA content of purified preparations of mouse Purkinje neurons isolated by a velocity sedimentation technique. *J. Neurochem., 20*, 651-657.

[36] Coggeshall, R. E. (1967). A light and electron microscope study of the abdominal ganglion of *Aplysia californica. J. Neurophysiol., 30*, 1263-1287.

[37] Coggeshall, R. E. (1972). Autoradiographic and chemical location of 5-Hydroxytryptamine in identified neurons in the leech. *Anat. Rec., 172*, 489-498.

[38] Coggeshall, R. E, Yaksta, B. A. & Swartz, F. J. (1970). A cytophotometric analysis of the DNA in the nucleus of the giant cell, R-2, in *Aplysia. Chromosoma, 32*, 205-212.

[39] Cuoghi, B. (2001). Glial cells: basic components of clusters of supramedullary neurons in pufferfishes. *J. Neurocytol., 30*, 503-513.

[40] Cuoghi, B. & Marini, M. (2001). Ultrastructural and cytochemical features of the supramedullary neurons of the pufferfish *Diodon holacanthus* (L.) (Osteichthyes). *Tissue Cell, 33*, 491-499.

[41] Cuoghi, B., Marini, M. & Mola, L. (2002). Histochemical and immunohistochemical localization of nitric oxide synthase in the supramedullary neurons of the pufferfish *Tetraodon fluviatilis. Brain Res., 938*, 3-6.

[42] Cuoghi, B., Blasiol, L. & Sabatini, M. A. (2003). ACTH occurrence in teleosts supramedullary neuron clusters: a neuron-glial common language ? *Gen. Comp. Endocrinol., 132*, 88-95.

[43] Dahmann, C., Diffley, J.F. & Nasmyth, K.A. (1995). S-phase-promoting cyclin-dependent kinases prevent re-replication by inhibiting the transition of replication origins to a pre-replicative state. *Curr. Biol., 5*, 1257-1269.

[44] Edgar, B. A. & Lehner, C. F. (1996). Developmental Control of Cell Cycle Regulators: A Fly's Perspective. *Science, 274*, 1646-1652.

[45] Edgar, B. A. & Orr-Weaver, T. L. (2001). Endoreplication Cell Cycles: More for Less. *Cell, 105*, 297-306.

[46] Frazier, W. T., Kandel E. R., Kupfermann, I. & Coggeshall R. E. (1967). Morphological and functional properties of identified neurons in the abdominal ganglion of *Aplysia californica. J. Neurophysiol., 30*, 1288-1351.

[47] Fritsch, G. (1886). Ueber einige bemerkenswerhe elemente des central nerven system von *Lophius piscatorius. Arch. Mikr. NAT. Entw.-Meech., 27*, 13-31.

[48] Fujita, S. (1973). DNA cytofluorimetry on large and small cell nuclei stained with pararosaniline Feulgen. *Histochimie, 36*, 193-199.

[49] Fujita, S. (1974). DNA constancy in neurons of human cerebellum and spinal cord as revealed by Feulgen cytofluorimetry and cytofluorimetry. *J. Comp. Neurol., 155*, 195-202.

[50] Fujita, S., Fukuda, M., Kitamura, T. & Yoshida, S. (1972). Two wave-length-scanning method in Feulgen cytophotometry. *Acta Histochem. Cytochem., 5*, 146-152.

[51] Fujita, S., Hattori, T., Fukuda, M. & Kitamura, T. (1974). DNA contents in Purkinje cells and inner granule neurons in developing rat certebellum. *Dev. Growth Diff., 16*, 205-212.

[52] Fukuda, M., Bohm, N. & Fujita, S. (1978). DNA constancy in neurons of the rat and human cerebellum. *Progr. Histochem. Cytochem., 11*, 20-24.

[53] Funakoshi, K., Katoda, T., Atobe, Y., Nakamo, M., Goris, R. C. & Kishida, R. (1998). Gastrin/CCK-ergic innervation of cutaneous mucous gland by the supramedullary cells of the puffer fish *Takifugu niphobles. Neurosci. Lett., 258*, 171-174.

[54] Gallant, P., Shiio, Y., Cheng, P. F., Parkhurst, S. M. & Eisenman, R. N. (1996). Myc and Max homologs in *Drosophila. Science, 274*, 1523-1527.

[55] Gaskell, J. F. (1919). Adrenalin in annelids. *J. Physiol., 2*, 73-85.

[56] Gerbi, S. A. & Urnov, F. D. (1996). Differential DNA replication in insects, In M. L. DePamphilis (Ed.), *DNA replication in eukaryotic cells* (pp. 947-969). Cold Spring Harbor, N.Y, USA: Cold Spring Harbor Laboratory Press.

[57] Giacometti, S., Scherini, E. & Bernocchi, G. (1986). Nuclear heterogeneity of the Purkinje neuron population in the cerebellum of the reptiles. *Boll. Zool., 53*, 359-364.

[58] Grandori, C., Cowley, S. M., James, L. P. & Eisenman, R. N. (2000). The Myc/Max/Mad network and the transcriptional control of cell behavior. *Ann. Rev. Cell Dev. Biol., 16*, 653-699.

[59] Hammond, M. P. & Laird, C. D. (1985). Chromosome structure and DNA replication in nurse and follicle cells of *Drosophila melanogaster. Chromosoma, 91*, 267-278.

[60] Heinz, E. (1944). Kleine Beitiage zur Zellenlehre II. Uber die Riesenkerne der Schneken und Asseln. *Rev. Suisse Zool., 51*, 402-404.

[61] Herman, C. J. & Lapham, L. W. (1968). DNA content of neurones in the cat hippocampus. *Science, 160*, 537.

[62] Herman, C. J. & Lapham, L. W. (1969). Neuronal polyploidy and nuclear volume in cat central nervous system. *Brain Res., 15*, 35-48.

[63] Hobi, R., Studer, M., Ruch, F. & Kuenzle, C. C. (1984). The DNA content of cerebral cortex neurons determinations by cytophotometry and high performance liquid chromatography. *Brain Res., 305*, 209-219.

[64] Kandel, E. R. (1976). *Cellular Basis of Behavior*. San Francisco, USA: Freeman & Co., p.221.

[65] Kowalska, E. & Marcinkowski, T. (1998). The amount of DNA in cells of the granular layer of the cerebellum and their susceptibility to hypoxia. *Med. Hypotheses, 51*, 443-444.

[66] Kuenzle, C. C., Bregrard, A., Hubschner, U. & Ruch, F. (1978). Extra DNA in forebrain neurons. *Exp. Cell Res., 113*, 151-160.

[67] Kunz, W. (1984). How genes are amplified in germ cells and somatic cells. In W. Engels (Ed.), *Advances in Invertebrate Reproduction*. (vol. III, pp. 65-71). New York, USA: Elsevier Press

[68] Laird, C. D. (1980). Structural paradox of polytene chromosomes. *Cell, 22*, 869-874.

[69] Lapham, L. W. (1965). The tetraploid DNA content of normal human Purkinje cells and its development during the perinatal period. A quantitative cytochemical study. *Excerpta Med. (Amst.) Cong. Ser., 100*, 445-449.

[70] Lapham, L. W. (1968). Tetraploid DNA content of purkinje neurones of human cerebellar cortex. *Science, 159*, 310-312.

[71] Lasek, R. J. & Dower, W. J. (1971). *Aplysia californica*: analysis of nuclear DNA in individual nuclei of giant neurons. *Science, 172*, 278-280.

[72] Lee, G. M., Rasch, E.M. & Thornthwaite, J. T. (1984). Cytophotometric comparisons of DNA levels in neuronal and glial cells of the cerebellum: a comparative study. *Cell Biochem. Funct., 2*, 225-236.

[73] Lentz, R. D. & Lapham, L. W. (1969). A quantitative cytochemical study of the DNA content of neurons of rat cerebellar cortex. *J. Neurochem., 16*, 379-384.

[74] Liang, C., Spitzer, J. D., Smith, H. S. & Gerbi, S. A. (1993). Replication initiates at a confined region during DNA amplification in *Sciara* DNA puff II/9A. *Genes Dev., 7*, 1072-1084.

[75] Lombardo, F. & Sonetti, D. (1977). The neuronal nuclei in the central ganglia of Planorbid snails. *The Nucleus, 20*, 271-277.

[76] Lombardo, F. & Sonetti, D. (1983). Amplification and under-replication of repetitive DNAs in the neuronal nuclei of *Planorbis corneus. Neurosci. Lett. Suppl., 14*, 226.

[77] Lombardo, F., Baraldi, E. & Sonetti, D. (1980). Differential staining and fluorescence of chromatin in population of neuronal nuclei from *Planorbis corneus. The Nucleus, 23*, 30-36.

[78] Manfredi Romanini, M. G., Fraschini, A. & Bernocchi, G. (1972). DNA content and nuclear area in the neurons of the cerebral ganglion in *Helix pomatia. Ann. Histochem., 18*, 49-58.

[79] Manicardi, G. C., Bizzaro, D., Sonetti, D., Lombardo, F. & Bianchi, U. (1992). Amplification of GC-rich DNAs in neuronal nuclei of *Planorbarius corneus* (L.) (Mollusca, Pulmonata). *Eur. J. Histochem., 36*, 303-309.

[80] Mann, D. M. A. & Yates, P. O. (1973). Polyploidy in the human nervous system. Part I. The DNA content of neurones and glia of the cerebellum. *J. Neurol. Sci., 18*, 183-196.

[81] Mann, D. M. A, Yates, P. O & Barton, C. M. (1978). The DNA content of Purkinje cells in mammals. *J. Comp. Neurol., 180*, 345-347.

[82] Manuelidis, L. & Manuelidis, E. E. (1974). On the DNA content of cerebellar Purkinje cells *in vivo* and *in vitro. Exp. Neurol., 43*, 192-206.

[83] Mares, V. & van-der-Ploeg, M. (1980). Cytophotometric re-investigation of DNA content in Purkinje cells of the rat cerebellum. *Histochemistry, 69*, 161-167.

[84] Mares, V., Lodin, Z. & Sacha, J. (1973). A cytochemical autoradiographic study of nuclear DNA in mouse Purkinje cells. *Brain Res., 53*, 273-289.

[85] Marini, M. & Benedetti, I. (1992). The Rohon-Beard cells and supramedullary neurons in Teleosts. In I. Benedetti, B. Bertolini & E. Capanna (Eds.), *Selected Symposia and monographs: Neurology today* (pp. 217-236). Modena, Italy: Mucchi.

[86] Marini, M., Benedetti, I. & Franchini, (1984). Ultrastructural features of supramedullary neurons in *Crenilabrus quinquemaculatus. Z. mikrosk-anat. Forsch, Leipzig, 98*, 63-71.

[87] Marshak, T. L., Mares, V. & Brodsky, V. Y. (1985). An attempt to influence DNA content in postmitotic Purkinje cells of the cerebellum. *Acta Histochem., 76*, 193-200.

[88] McIlwain, D. L. & Capps-Covey, P. (1976). The nuclear DNA content of large ventral spinal neurons. *J. Neurochem., 27*, 109-112.

[89] Mola, L. & Cuoghi, B. (2004). The supramedullary neurons of fish: present status and goals for the future. *Brain Res. Bull., 64*, 195-204.

[90] Mola, L., Marini, M. & Benedetti, I. (1992). Acid phosphatase activity in the supramedullary neurons of *Coris julis* (L.). *Eur. J. Histochem., 36*, 233-236.

[91] Mola, L., Cuoghi, B., Mandrioli, M. & Marini, M. (2001). DNA endoreplication in the clustered supramedullary neurons of the pufferfish *Diodon holacanthus* L. (Osteichthyes). *Histochem. J., 33*, 59-63.

[92] Mola, L., Sassi, D. & Cuoghi, B. (2002). The supramedullary cells of the teleost *Coris julis* (L.): a noradrenergic neuronal system. *Eur. J. Histochem., 46*, 329-332.

[93] Montarolo, P. G., Kandel, E. R. & Schacher, S. (1988). Long-term heterosynaptic inhibition in *Aplysia. Nature, 12*, 333, 171-174.

[94] Morselt, A. F. W., Braakman, D. J. & James, J. (1972). Feulgen-DNA and fast green histone estimation in individual cell nuclei of cerebellum of young and old rats. *Acta Histochem., 43*, 281-286.

[95] Nagata, Y., Muro, Y. & Todokoro, K. (1997). Thrombopoietin-induced polyploidization of bone marrow megakaryocytes is due to a unique regulatory mechanism in late mitosis. *J. Cell Biol., 139*, 449-457.

[96] Nakajima, Y., Pappas, G. D. & Bennett, M. V. L. (1965). The fine structure of the supramedullary neurons of the puffer with special reference to endocellular and pericellular capillaries. *Am. J. Anat., 116*, 471-492.

[97] Novaková, V., Sandritter, W. & Schlueter, G. (1970). DNA content of neurons in rat central nervous system. *Exp. Cell Res., 60*, 454-456.

[98] Orian, A., van Steensel, B., Delrow, J., Bussemaker, H. J., Li, L., Sawado, T., Williams, E., Loo, L. W., Cowley, S. M., Yost, C. (2003). Genomic binding by the *Drosophila* Myc, Max, Mad/Mnt transcription factor network. *Genes Dev. 17*, 1101–1114.

[99] Osborne, N. N. (1972). The *in vivo* synthesis of serotonin in an identified serotonin-containing neuron of *Helix pomatia. Int. J. Neurosci., 3*, 215-219.

[100] Osborne N. N. (1978). *Biochemistry of characterised neuron*. Oxford, UK: Pergamon Press.

[101] Osheim, Y. N. & Miller, O. L. Jr. (1983). Novel amplification and transcriptional activity of chorion genes in *Drosophila melanogaster* follicle cells. *Cell, 33*, 543-553.

[102] Pentreath, V. W., Berry, M. S. & Cottrell, G. A. (1974). Anatomy of the giant dopamine-containing neurone in the left pedal ganglion of *Planorbis corneus. Cell Tissue Res. 151*, 369-384.

[103] Picciotto, M. R., Johnshon, R. & Schellers, R. M. (1986). Neuropeptide genes are not selectively amplified in *Aplysia* polyploid neurons. *Neurol. Neurobiol., 20*, 429-434.

[104] Pierce, S. B., Yost B., Britton, J. S., Flynn, E. M., Edgar, B. A. & Eisenman, E. N. (2004). dMyc is required for larval growth and endoreplication in *Drosophila. Development, 131*, 2317-2327.

[105] Quattrini, D. (1950). Particolarità strutturali del nucleo di *Helix vermiculata* Muller. *Rend. Acc. Naz. Lincei (ser. VIII), 8*, 149-152.

[106] Roberts, J. M., Buck, L. B. & Axel, R. (1983). A structure for amplified DNA, *Cell, 33*, 53-63.

[107] Sandritter, W., Novaková, V., Pilny, J. & Kiefer, G. (1967). Cytophotometrische Messungen des Nuklein-Saure und Proteingehaltes von Ganglienzellen der Ratte wahrend der postnatalen Entwicklung und im Alter. *Z. Zellforsch., 80*, 145-152.

[108] Sassi, D., Manicardi, G. C., Mola, L. & Benedetti, I. (1995). Cytofluorimetric evidence for differential genome endoreplication in the cluster neurons of *Lophius piscatorius* L. (Osteichthyes, Lophiiformes). *Eur. J. Histochem., 39*, 117-126.

[109] Sauer, K., Knoblich, J.A., Richardson, H. & Lehner, C.F. (1995). Distinct modes of cyclin E/cdc2c kinase regulation and S-phase control in mitotic and endoreduplication cycles of *Drosophila* embryogenesis. *Genes Dev., 9*, 1327-1339.

[110] Schwob, E., Bohm, T., Mendenhall, M.D. & Nasmyth, K. (1994). The B-type cyclin kinase inhibitor p40SIC1 controls the G1 to S transition in *S. cerevisiae*. *Cell*, 79, 233-244.

[111] Sinclair, J. H. & Brown, D. D. (1971). Retention of common nucleotide sequences in the ribosomal deoxyribonucleic acid of eukaryotes and some of their physical characteristics. *Biochemistry, 10*, 2761-2769.

[112] Smith, A.V. & Orr-Weaver, T.L. (1991). The regulation of the cell cycle during *Drosophila* embryogenesis: the transition to polyteny. *Development, 112*, 997-1008.

[113] Sonetti, D. & Peruzzi, E. (2004). Neuron-microglia communication in the CNS of the freshwater snail *Planorbarius corneus*. *Acta Biol. Hung., 55*, 273-285.

[114] Sonetti, D., Lusvardi, C. & Fasolo, A. (1990). Immunohistochemical localization of some vertebrate neuropeptides (SP, NPY, CGRP, CCK8) in the central nervous system of the freshwater snail *Planorbarius corneus*. *Cell Tissue Res., 260*, 435-448.

[115] Sonetti, D., Peruzzi, E. & Stefano, G. B. (2005). Endogenous morphine and ACTH association in neural tissues. *Med. Sci. Monit. 11*, MS22-30.

[116] Spradling, A.C. (1981). The organization and amplification of two chromosomal domains containing *Drosophila* chorion genes. *Cell, 27*, 193-201.

[117] Stefano, G. B. & Sharrer, B. (1994). Endogenous morphine and related opiates, a new class of chemical messengers. *Adv. Neuroimmunol., 4*, 57-68.

[118] Swartz, F. J. & Bhatnagar, K. P. (1981). Are CNS neurons polyploid? A critical analysis based upon cytophotometric study of the DNA content of cerebellar and olfactory bulbar neurons of the bat. *Brain Res., 208*, 267-281.

[119] Tollervey, D., Lehtonen, H., Jansen, R., Kern, H. & Hurt, E. C. (1993). Temperature-sensitive mutations demonstrate roles for yeast fibrillarin in pre-rRNA processing, pre-rRNA methylation, and ribosome assembly. *Cell, 72*, 443-457.

[120] Traas, J., Hülskamp, M., Gendreau, E. & Höfte, H. (1998). Endoreplication and development: rule without dividing? *Curr. Opin. Plant Biol., 1*, 498-503.

[121] Urata, Y., Parmelee, S. J., Agard, D. A. & Sedat, J. W. (1995). A three-dimensional structural dissection of *Drosophila* polytene chromosomes. *J. Cell Biol., 131*, 279-295.

[122] Van der Wilt, G. J., Roest, M. & Janse, C. (1987). Neuronal substrates of respiratory behavior and related functions in *Lymnaea stagnalis*. In H. H Boer, W. P. M. Geraerts & J. Joosse J. (Eds.), *Proceedings of the second symposium on molluscan neurobiology: Neurobiology, Molluscan models* (pp. 292-296). Amsterdam, The Netherlands: North Holland publ. Co.

[123] Varmuza, S., Prideaux, V., Kothary, R. & Rossant, J. (1988). Polytene chromosomes in mouse trophoblast giant cells. *Development, 102*, 127-134.

[124] White, M. J. D. (1973). *Animal Cytology and Evolution.* (Third Edition). Cambridge, UK: Cambridge University Press.

[125] Zimmet, J. & Ravid, K. (2000). Polyploidy: occurrence in nature, mechanisms, and significance for the megakaryocyte-platelet system. *Exp. Hematol., 28*: 3-16.

[126] Zhou, Z. Q. & Hurlin, P. J. (2001). The interplay between Mad and Myc in proliferation and differentiation. *Trends Cell Biol., 11*, S10-S14.

[127] Zottoli, S. J., Akanki, F. R., Hiza, N. A., Ho-Sang, Jr, D. A., Motta, M., Tan, X. & Watts K. M. (1999). Physiological characterization of supramedullary/dorsal neurons of the cunner *Tautogolabrus adspersus*. *Biol. Bull., 197*, 239-240.

[128] Zottoli, S. J., Arnolds, D. E. W., Asamoah, N. O., Chenez, C., Fuller, S. N., Hiza, N., A. & Nierman, J. E. (2001). Dye coupling evidence for gap junctions between supramedullary neurons of the cunner *Tautogolabrus adspersus. Biol. Bull., 201,* 277-278.

[129] Zybina, E. V. & Zybina, T. G. (1996). Polytene chromosomes in mammalian cells. *Int. Rev. Cytol., 165,* 53-119.

In: New Trends in Brain Research
Editor: F. J. Chen, pp. 61-74

ISBN 1-59454-834-X
© 2006 Nova Science Publishers, Inc.

Chapter III

ENDOPLASMIC RETICULUM STRESS-INDUCED APOPTOSIS AND ITS PREVENTION BY NEUROTROPHINS

Koji Shimoke and *Toshihiko Ikeuchi*

Laboratory of Neurobiology, Faculty of Engineering and High Technology Research Center (HRC), Kansai University, 3-3-35 Yamate-cho, Suita, Osaka 564-8680, Japan

ABSTRACT

Recently, some genes responsible for neuronal degenerative disorders such as Alzheimer's disease and Parkinson's disease have been identified, and detailed analyses of the molecular mechanisms underlying the onset of neurodegenerative diseases have been carried out. In addition to genetic effectors, environmental effectors acting on cellular homeostatic controls have been analyzed at the molecular level. From these analyses, it has been revealed that endoplasmic reticulum (ER) stress, which is caused by the accumulation of unfolded proteins in the ER, is closely involved in the onset of neurodegenerative processes in neurons. On the other hand, it has also been revealed that neurons die through apoptotic cell death during neurodegenerative processes. However, the molecular mechanism by which ER stress induces apoptosis in neurons remains unclear. In addition, the molecular mechanism behind the processes protecting against ER stress-induced apoptosis in neurons has not been elucidated. We have recently reported that neurotrophins including NGF (nerve growth factor) and BDNF (brain-derived neurotrophic factor) can suppress ER stress-induced apoptosis in PC12 cells as a model of neurons and in cultured cerebral cortical neurons, respectively. Here we review the intracellular signaling mechanism by which neurotrophins prevent ER stress-induced apoptosis in neuronal cells.

* Address correspondence to: Dr. K. Shimoke, Laboratory of Neurobiology, Faculty of Engineering and High Technology Research Center (HRC), Kansai University, 3-3-35 Yamate-cho, Suita, Osaka 564-8680, Japan. Tel: +81-6-6368-0853, Fax: +81-6-6330-3770; E-mail: shimoke@ipcku.kansai-u.ac.jp

INTRODUCTION

As the organ controlling the homeostatic balance of higher organisms, the brain has multiple functions. These functions are strictly regulated by neurons and glial cells in the brain. However, the brain is one of the most labile organs in higher organisms. If the control system in the brain breaks down, the homeostatic balance can not be maintained and serious symptoms arise. In humans, learning and memory are highly developed. Therefore, humans have been able to construct the most advanced society on the earth by employing their brain functions. As the average life span of humans continues to increase, medical care for senior citizens is more and more essential to society. In particular, therapeutic treatments for neuronal degenerative diseases such as Alzheimer's and Parkinson's diseases are very important, because most patients with such diseases need care and also therapeutic treatments. Basically, these diseases are closely related to the quality of life (QOL) of senior citizens.

Some neurons of patients with neurodegenerative diseases are considered to be exposed to ER stress and consequently undergo apoptotic cell death [14,18-20,23,26,30,39,42]. The sources of ER stress are genetic or acquired after birth. Whether ER stress is induced by genetic or acquired effectors, neurons die through apoptotic signaling specific to ER stress, and not through ordinary apoptotic signaling [14,36,38]. On the other hand, neurotrophins including NGF (nerve growth factor) and BDNF (brain-derived neurotrophic factor) are known to suppress ordinary apoptosis [3,16,51]. It is of interest whether neurotrophins can also suppress ER stress-specific apoptosis or not. In this article, we describe the intracellular apoptotic signaling mechanism by which ER stress induces neuronal death, and also the protective signaling mechanism by which neurotrophins suppress ER stress-induced apoptosis, in PC12 cells as a model neuron and primary cultured cerebral cortical neurons.

NEURODEGENERATIVE DISEASES AND APOPTOSIS

Apoptosis is physiologically essential for the developmental processes of vertebrates. In neuronal development, neurons are produced in duplicate, but half die through apoptosis before birth [40]. This process is considered a mechanism to eliminate incorrect synaptic connections produced during neuronal development. On the other hand, apoptosis is closely involved in neurodegenerative diseases. Some specific neurons of patients with neurodegenerative diseases are known to die through the apoptotic process [18-20,23,26,30,39,42]. The causes of neurodegenerative diseases include genetic and environmental factors, and the intracellular signaling mechanisms by which specific neurons die through apoptosis have gradually been elucidated. Along with these findings, specific genes responsible for a number of neurodegenerative diseases have been identified [5]. In the case of Alzheimer's disease, hippocampal neurons die through apoptosis and then basal forebrain cholinergic neurons projecting to the hippocampus also die through apoptosis, affecting learning, memory and behavior. The responsible genes involve those encoding amyloid precursor protein (APP) [4,10], presenilin 1 (PS1) [24,48] and presenilin 2 (PS2) [32]. And the apolipoprotein E (apoE) gene is considered a risk factor for Alzheimer's disease [33,59]. In the case of Parkinson's disease, dopaminergic neurons of the substantia nigra undergo apoptotic cell death, resulting in loss of motional control, because these neurons project to the striatum. The parkin and chip genes have been identified as responsible for the disease [17,18,27]. In the case of Huntington's disease, neurons of the striatum undergo apoptosis, resulting in loss of motional and behavioral control. The huntingtin gene is known as the gene responsible for the disease [45].

Typically in apoptosis, following the production of reactive oxygen species (ROS) and mitochondrial dysfunction, a cascade of several caspases, which are serine proteases, is activated (Figure 1) [1,7,12,31,44]. The caspase cascade eventually activates caspase-3-activated DNase (CAD), and then the fragmentation of chromosomal DNA and condensation of the nucleus occur, resulting in apoptotic death [8]. Therefore, it has been believed that neurons of patients with neurodegenerative diseases die through ordinary apoptosis, during which the cytochrome c released from injured mitochondria forms an apoptosome with pro-caspase-9, dATP and Apaf-1, the apoptosome activates caspase-9 (initiator caspase), activated caspase-9 activates caspase-3 (executioner caspase), activated caspase-3 activates CAD, and then activated CAD cleaves chromosomal DNA (Figure 1) [1,8]. In ordinary apoptosis, it is also known that pro-apoptotic Bcl-2 family proteins are involved [46,58].

ER STRESS-INDUCED APOPTOSIS

Recently, the apoptosis of neurons in neurodegenerative diseases has been revealed as different from the ordinary apoptosis mentioned above, whether caused by genetic or environmental factors. It has been observed that unfolded proteins are accumulated in the endoplasmic reticulum (ER) of neurons in neurodegenerative diseases [35,42]. This type of stress is known as ER stress. ER stress also causes apoptosis of neurons. In cultured cells, ER stress is easily induced by the addition of inhibitors of protein glycosylation in the ER [49,53], inhibitors of Ca^{2+} ATPase on the ER [28,34,47], or inhibitors on protein transport from the ER to the golgi apparatus [2]. It has been reported that during ER stress-induced apoptosis of rat or mouse neurons, caspase-12 in the ER is specifically activated [38]. On the other hand, caspase-4, which is also located in the ER, is

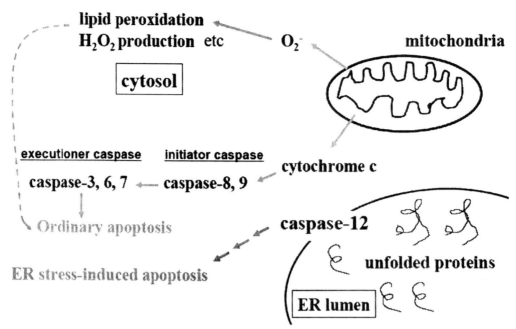

Figure 1. Signaling pathways during ordinary apoptosis and ER stress-induced apoptosis. In ordinary apoptosis, initiator caspases (caspase-8 or -9) are activated by the formation of an apoptosome containing cytochrome c released from mitochondria, pro-caspase-9, dATP and Apaf-1. These caspases activate executioner caspases (caspase-3, -6, or -7) by the proteolytic cleavage of their pro-forms. In ER stress-induced apoptosis, caspase-12 on the ER membrane is activated by the accumulation of unfolded proteins in the ER lumen. The signaling pathways are indicated by green arrows for ordinary apoptosis and by red arrows for ER stress-induced apoptosis.

similarly activated during ER stress-induced apoptosis of human neurons [14]. After the activation of caspase-12, caspase-9 is activated without the release of cytochrome c from mitochondria (Figure 2), and then the caspase cascade downstream of caspase-9 is activated as in ordinary apoptosis [1]. We also observed similar apoptotic signaling during ER stress-induced apoptosis in cultured cerebral cortical neurons and PC12 cells [49,53]. Therefore, there exist two apoptotic signalings, ordinary apoptotic signaling and the ER stress-induced apoptotic signaling (Figure 1). In order to investigate the relation between mitochondrial dysfunction and ER stress-induced apoptotic signaling, we performed the following experiments. 1-Methyl-4-phenyl-1,2,3,6-tetrahydropyridine (MPTP), an inducer of a model of Parkinson's disease, is converted to active MPP^+ by MAO-B [50,52]. Because MPP^+ induces the apoptosis of dopaminergic neurons in substantia nigra, MPTP is widely used in fundamental research on Parkinson's disease. We treated PC12 cells with MPTP or MPP^+, and monitored the induction of expression of glucose-regulated protein 78 (GRP78) as a marker of ER stress. It was found that although MPTP induced apoptotic death in PC12 cells, the expression of GRP78 was not induced [52]. Interestingly, however, peroxides (lipid peroxides) were produced through mitochondrial dysfunction, and caspase-3 was activated time-dependently after the treatment with MPTP [52]. These results indicate that MPTP induces ordinary

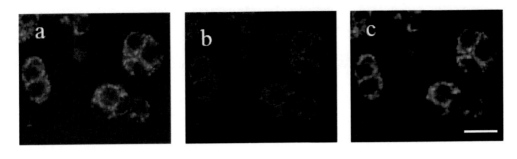

| Cytochrome c | Mito Tracker | Merge |

Figure 2. Cytochrome c is not released from mitochondria during ER stress-induced apoptosis.
To induce ER stress, PC12 cells were cultured for 24 hours with 1 µg/ml of tunicamycin. Then, cells were fixed and permeated for immunocytostaining with anti-cytochrome c antibody (a). At the same time, cells were treated with MitoTrackerRed to stain mitochondria (b). A merged image of a and b is indicated (c). Bar denotes 30 µm.

apoptosis dependent on mitochondrial dysfunction, but does not induce the ER stress-mediated apoptosis independent of mitochondrial dysfunction. Thus, mitochondrial pathway involved in ordinary apoptosis is not important for ER stress-mediated apoptosis. This notion is supported by the analysis using APAF1$^{-/-}$ cells [43]. Furthermore, it is known that some pro-apoptotic Bcl-2 family proteins are also involved in ER stress-mediated apoptosis [6,37,47]. In these reports, a dependency of the mitochondrial pathway is suggested. Thus, we think that further analyses are needed to understand total mechanisms of ER stress-mediated apoptosis.

ENDOGENOUS PROTECTION MECHANISMS AGAINST ER STRESS

When cells are exposed to ER stress, several endogenous protection mechanisms are known to be activated. For example, the induction of expression of molecular chaperons including GRP78 and GRP94, and the abeyance of de novo protein synthesis occurs through the activation of sensor proteins including Ire1α, PERK and ATF6 by unfolded proteins accumulated in the ER lumen (Figure 3) [25,35,42,56]. Recently, OASIS, which acts specifically in astrocytes, has been identified as a new sensor protein for the expression of GRP78 [29]. This protective mechanism is referred to as the unfolded protein response (UPR). Ireβ and PERK also inhibit the biosynthesis of a protein by cleaving 28S rRNA and by phosphorylating eIF2α to prevent further accumulation of unfolded proteins in the ER (Figure 3). Another known mechanism of protection is the system of endoplasmic reticulum-associated degradation (ERAD), which degradates unfolded proteins by the ubiquitin-proteasome pathway after excreting them from the ER lumen through p97/ valosin-containing protein (VCP) (Figure 4) [9,13]. To examine whether NGF enhances the degradation of unfolded proteins by the ubiquitin-proteasome pathway or not, we measured the proteasome activity in PC12 cells with or without the NGF treatment. The proteasome activity in NGF-treated PC12 cells was not significantly changed from that in untreated cells [unpublished data], suggesting that NGF suppresses ER stress-induced apoptosis by inhibiting the activation of the caspase cascade, not by inhibiting the ER stress itself or by enhancing the ERAD endogenous protection mechanism. Interestingly, it is also known that UPR is a mediator of ER stress-induced apoptosis via Ire1, PERK and ATF6 [26]. This discrepancy of UPR function is not elucidated, however, it is reported that there are detailed molecular mechanisms of UPR as a mediator of ER stress-induced apoptosis [26].

Fig.3

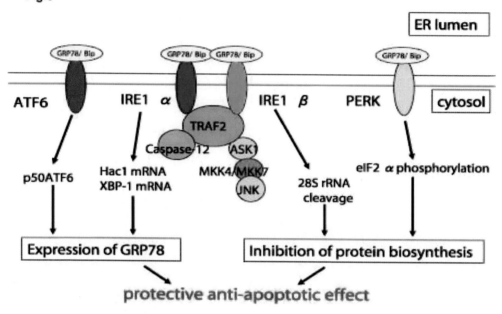

Figure 3. Endogenous protection mechanisms against ER stress. Four sensor proteins (ATF6, Ire1α, Ire1β and PERK) for ER stress have been identified, and their functions are indicated. ATF6 and Ire1α induce the expression of GRP78 through binding to cis-element (UPRE) of cleaved ATF6 and XBP-1 protein, respectively. Ire1β and PERK inhibit protein biosynthesis by the cleavage of 28S rRNA and the phosphorylation of eIF2α, respectively. As a result, ER stress and the subsequent apoptosis are attenuated.

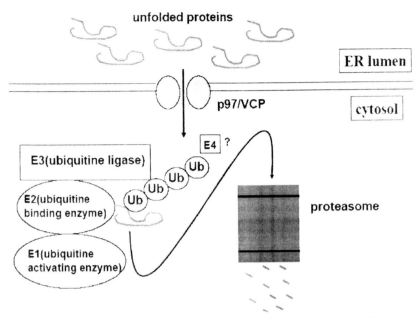

Figure 4. Prevention of ER stress via the ERAD system. Unfolded proteins are eliminated from the ER lumen through p97/VCP and are polyubiquitinated by E1, E2, E3 and E4. Polyubiquitinated unfolded proteins are specifically trapped by the proteasome and degradated into amino acids.

NEUROTROPHINS AND THEIR FUNCTIONS

Neurotrophins including nerve growth factor (NGF), brain-derived neurotrophic factor (BDNF), neurotrophin-3 (NT-3) and neurotrophin-4/5 (NT-4/5) are a family of neurotrophic factors acting on neurons as differentiation- and survival-promoting factors and modulators of synaptic plasticity [3,22]. The Trk family comprising TrkA, TrkB and TrkC are membrane-spanning receptors on the cell membrane of neurons. TrkA, TrkB and TrkC are the specific receptors for NGF, BDNF plus NT-4/5, and NT-3, respectively (Figure 5) [21,41]. When these receptors are activated by the binding of specific ligands, several tyrosine residues are autophosphorylated in their intracellular regions. The actions of the neurotrophins mentioned above are achieved by the binding of specific signaling proteins to specific sites surrounding the phosphorylated tyrosines in the intracellular regions of TrkA, TrkB and TrkC. Then, the bound signaling proteins are also phosphorylated by Trk receptors, and transmit the neurotrophin signal to downstream signaling proteins [21,22,41]. The downstream signaling pathways contain several protein phosphorylation cascades. At least three signaling pathways have been discovered downstream of Trk receptors. They are the Ras/mitogen-activated protein kinase (MAPK) pathway, the phosphatidylinositol 3-kinase (PI3-K)/Akt pathway, and the PLC-gamma pathway (Figure 5) [11,15,55,57]. We have already found that neurotrophins can protect against ordinary apoptosis through the PI3-K/Akt pathway in low K$^-$-treated cultured cerebellar granule neurons [51,54] and in MPTP-treated PC12 cells [50]. As the typical anti-apoptotic signaling pathway, the PI3-K/Akt pathway is known to protect a number of neurons from the ordinary apoptosis induced by various stimulants. Akt in the PI3-K/Akt pathway phosphorylates and inhibits pro-apoptotic proteins including BAD, pro-caspase-9, forkhead transcription factor (FKHR) and inhibitor NF-kappaB kinase (IKK), leading to the suppression of ordinary apoptosis [16, see introduction of 49].

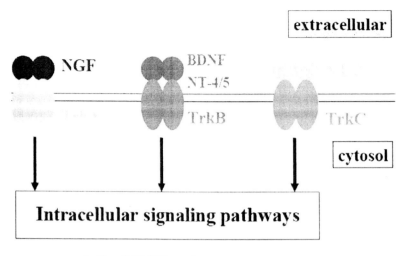

Figure 5. Neurotrophins and their receptors. Neurotrophins (NGF, BDNF, NT-3 and NT-4/5) are divided into three groups by the specificity of their receptor binding. NGF, BDNF plus NT-4/5, and NT-3 bind to TrkA, TrkB, and TrkC, respectively, on the cell membrane. Upon the binding of neurotrophins, intracellular regions of TrkA, TrkB and TrkC are phosphorylated and activated, and then intracellular signaling pathways including many kinases are activated. The common major pathways are the Ras/mitogen-activated protein kinase (MAPK) pathway, the phosphatidylinositol 3-kinase/Akt pathway, and the phospholipase C-gamma pathway.

SUPPRESSION OF ER STRESS-INDUCED APOPTOSIS BY NEUROTROPHINS

We found that neurotrophins can also suppress the ER stress-induced apoptosis in neurons treated with tunicamycin, an inhibitor of the glycosylation of newly synthesized proteins [49,53]. During the progression of ER stress-induced apoptosis, caspase-12, the ER stress-specific caspase, is known to be activated [38]. Then, we considered that the activation of caspase-12 could be suppressed by the PI3-K/Akt pathway triggered by neurotrophins, leading to the suppression of the ER stress-mediated apoptosis. Therefore, we measured the activity of caspase-12 in tunicamycin-treated cerebral cortical neurons and PC12 cells with or without the addition of BDNF and NGF, respectively. BDNF and NGF significantly suppressed the activation of caspase-12. In the presence of LY294002, a specific inhibitor of PI3-K, no suppression of the activation of caspase-12 by BDNF and NGF was observed. In addition, the PI3-K/Akt pathway triggered by BDNF and NGF also suppressed the activation of caspase-9 and caspase-3. It has been reported that caspase-12 directly activates caspase-9 which in turn activates caspase-3 [36]. These results indicate that the ER stress-induced apoptotic signaling initiated by the activation of caspase-12 proceeds to the activation of caspase-9 and the activation of caspase-3, and then executes the death process, in cultured cerebral cortical neurons and PC12 cells (Figure 6). The fact that similar results were obtained in both cerebral cortical neurons and PC12 cells suggests the presence of a common intracellular signal transduction mechanism in both cells. In addition, we suggest that the anti-apoptotic effect of BDNF and NGF on the caspase cascade is achieved by the inhibition of an unknown effector acting as the activator of caspase-12 in the pathway upstream of the caspase cascade (Figure 6). We consider that one should identify the effector X and search for its suppressor, because the amino acid sequence of pro-caspase-12 does not contain the sequence recognized by Akt.

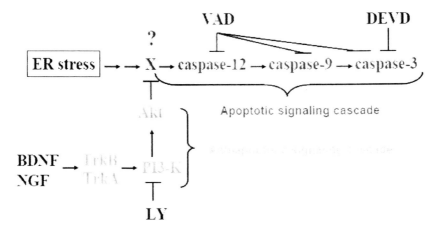

Figure 6. **A proposed model for the signaling pathway of the anti-apoptotic effect of BDNF and NGF on ER stress-induced apoptosis**. ER stress is initiated by treatment with tunicamycin. Caspase-12 is activated by the unknown effector protein X in the apoptotic signaling induced by tunicamycin. Activated caspase-12 directly cleaves pro-caspase-9 and produces an active caspase-9 in the process of ER stress-induced apoptosis. Then, activated caspase-9 cleaves pro-caspase-3 as in ordinary apoptosis. On the other hand, neurotrophins (NGF and BDNF) bind to their receptors and induce anti-apoptotic signaling to activate downstream kinases. Activated Akt may phosphorylate the unknown effector X to suppress the activation of caspase-12 and ER stress-induced apoptosis. The actions of a general inhibitor of caspases (VAD), a specific inhibitor of caspase-3 (DEVD), and a specific inhibitor of PI3-K (LY) (LY294002) are also indicated.

ENDOCRINE-DISRUPTING MATERIALS INDUCE ER STRESS AND ER STRESS-MEDIATED APOPTOSIS

Recently, reports about the effects of endocrine-disrupting materials on human germ cells have provided warnings of the dangers such materials rose as water pollutants affecting future generations. However, there have been few reports about their effects on neuronal cells. We have been investigating the effects of endocrine-disrupting materials on PC12 cells, and found that some activate caspase-12 and induce ER stress-mediated apoptosis [unpublished data]. We are examining the relation between the pro-apoptotic effect of endocrine-disrupting materials and some neurodegenerative diseases.

CONCLUSION

It has been reported that caspase-12 is activated by ER stress, however, the mechanism behind the activation is yet to be completely clarified. Nakagawa et al. have reported that calpain, which is activated by calcium ion, is involved in the activation of caspase-12. Tunicamycin, an inhibitor of protein glycosylation in the ER, releases only a small amount of calcium ion from ER, suggesting that calcium ion is not an exclusive activator for caspase-12. Therefore, we consider that a detailed analysis of how the complex containing TRAF2, which binds to Ire1, activates caspase-12 is important to elucidate the mechanism of activation of caspase-12. We expect human caspase-4, the human homologue of caspase-12, to become a target in therapeutic studies.

Because no decisive strategy for the therapeutic treatment of neurodegenerative diseases has yet been established, many fundamental studies to protect neurons against apoptosis have been undertaken. Although applicative studies of neurotrophins have also been carried out to develop drugs and to exploit gene therapy, the efficacy of neurotrophins as a drug for neurodegenerative diseases has not yet been established. We consider that we should identify signaling proteins acting in the apoptotic pathway triggered by ER stress and in the preventive pathway activated by neurotrophins, and aim at drug design and gene therapy targeting these signaling proteins. Although most studies on the therapeutic treatment of neurodegenerative diseases have focused on those caused by genetic factors, most neurodegenerative diseases are caused by environmental factors. Because the PI3-K/Akt pathway is thought to be important to neurodegenerative diseases caused by genetic and environmental factors, further fundamental studies on PI3-K/Akt signaling are necessary.

REFERENCES

[1]   Adams, J.M. and Cory, S., Apoptosomes: engines for caspase activation, *Curr Opin Cell Biol*, 14 (2002) 715-20.
[2]   Aoki, S., Su, Q., Li, H., Nishikawa, K., Ayukawa, K., Hara, Y., Namikawa, K., Kiryu-Seo, S., Kiyama, H. and Wada, K., Identification of an axotomy-induced glycosylated protein, AIGP1, possibly involved in cell death triggered by endoplasmic reticulum-Golgi stress, *J Neurosci*, 22 (2002) 10751-60.
[3]   Barde, Y.A., Trophic factors and neuronal survival, *Neuron*, 2 (1989) 1525-34.
[4]   Chartier-Harlin, M.C., Crawford, F., Houlden, H., Warren, A., Hughes, D., Fidani, L., Goate, A., Rossor, M., Roques, P., Hardy, J. and et al., Early-onset Alzheimer's disease caused by mutations at codon 717 of the beta-amyloid precursor protein gene, *Nature*, 353 (1991) 844-6.
[5]   Cruts, M. and Van Broeckhoven, C., Molecular genetics of Alzheimer's disease, *Ann Med*, 30 (1998) 560-5.
[6]   Elyaman, W., Terro, F., Suen, K.C., Yardin, C., Chang, R.C. and Hugon, J., BAD and Bcl-2 regulation are early events linking neuronal endoplasmic reticulum stress to mitochondria-mediated apoptosis, *Brain Res Mol Brain Res*, 109 (2002) 233-8.
[7]   Emerit, J., Edeas, M. and Bricaire, F., Neurodegenerative diseases and oxidative stress, *Biomed Pharmacother*, 58 (2004) 39-46.

[8]   Enari, M., Sakahira, H., Yokoyama, H., Okawa, K., Iwamatsu, A. and Nagata, S., A caspase-activated DNase that degrades DNA during apoptosis, and its inhibitor ICAD, *Nature*, 391 (1998) 43-50.

[9]   Friedlander, R., Jarosch, E., Urban, J., Volkwein, C. and Sommer, T., A regulatory link between ER-associated protein degradation and the unfolded-protein response, *Nat Cell Biol*, 2 (2000) 379-84.

[10]   Goate, A., Chartier-Harlin, M.C., Mullan, M., Brown, J., Crawford, F., Fidani, L., Giuffra, L., Haynes, A., Irving, N., James, L. and et al., Segregation of a missense mutation in the amyloid precursor protein gene with familial Alzheimer's disease, *Nature*, 349 (1991) 704-6.

[11]   Gomez, N. and Cohen, P., Dissection of the protein kinase cascade by which nerve growth factor activates MAP kinases, *Nature*, 353 (1991) 170-3.

[12]   Green, D.R. and Reed, J.C., Mitochondria and apoptosis, *Science*, 281 (1998) 1309-12.

[13]   Hershko, A. and Ciechanover, A., The ubiquitin system, *Annu Rev Biochem*, 67 (1998) 425-79.

[14]   Hitomi, J., Katayama, T., Eguchi, Y., Kudo, T., Taniguchi, M., Koyama, Y., Manabe, T., Yamagishi, S., Bando, Y., Imaizumi, K., Tsujimoto, Y. and Tohyama, M., Involvement of caspase-4 in endoplasmic reticulum stress-induced apoptosis and Abeta-induced cell death, *J Cell Biol*, 165 (2004) 347-56.

[15]   Holgado-Madruga, M., Moscatello, D.K., Emlet, D.R., Dieterich, R. and Wong, A.J., Grb2-associated binder-1 mediates phosphatidylinositol 3-kinase activation and the promotion of cell survival by nerve growth factor, *Proc Natl Acad Sci U S A*, 94 (1997) 12419-24.

[16]   Ikeuchi, T., Shimoke, K., Kubo, T., Yamada, M. and Hatanaka, H., [Apoptosis-inducing and -preventing signal transduction pathways in cultured cerebellar granule neurons], *Hum Cell*, 11 (1998) 125-40.

[17]   Imai, Y., Soda, M., Hatakeyama, S., Akagi, T., Hashikawa, T., Nakayama, K.I. and Takahashi, R., CHIP is associated with Parkin, a gene responsible for familial Parkinson's disease, and enhances its ubiquitin ligase activity, *Mol Cell*, 10 (2002) 55-67.

[18]   Imai, Y., Soda, M., Inoue, H., Hattori, N., Mizuno, Y. and Takahashi, R., An unfolded putative transmembrane polypeptide, which can lead to endoplasmic reticulum stress, is a substrate of Parkin, *Cell*, 105 (2001) 891-902.

[19]   Jakobsen, L.D. and Jensen, P.H., Parkinson's disease: alpha-synuclein and parkin in protein aggregation and the reversal of unfolded protein stress, *Methods Mol Biol*, 232 (2003) 57-66.

[20]   Jellinger, K.A., Recent developments in the pathology of Parkinson's disease, *J Neural Transm Suppl* (2002) 347-76.

[21]   Kaplan, D.R. and Miller, F.D., Signal transduction by the neurotrophin receptors, *Curr Opin Cell Biol*, 9 (1997) 213-21.

[22]   Kaplan, D.R. and Miller, F.D., Neurotrophin signal transduction in the nervous system, *Curr Opin Neurobiol*, 10 (2000) 381-91.

[23]   Katayama, T., Imaizumi, K., Manabe, T., Hitomi, J., Kudo, T. and Tohyama, M., Induction of neuronal death by ER stress in Alzheimer's disease, *J Chem Neuroanat*, 28 (2004) 67-78.

[24] Katayama, T., Imaizumi, K., Sato, N., Miyoshi, K., Kudo, T., Hitomi, J., Morihara, T., Yoneda, T., Gomi, F., Mori, Y., Nakano, Y., Takeda, J., Tsuda, T., Itoyama, Y., Murayama, O., Takashima, A., St George-Hyslop, P., Takeda, M. and Tohyama, M., Presenilin-1 mutations downregulate the signalling pathway of the unfolded-protein response, *Nat Cell Biol*, 1 (1999) 479-85.

[25] Kaufman, R.J., Stress signaling from the lumen of the endoplasmic reticulum: coordination of gene transcriptional and translational controls, *Genes Dev*, 13 (1999) 1211-33.

[26] Kaufman, R.J., Orchestrating the unfolded protein response in health and disease, *J Clin Invest*, 110 (2002) 1389-98.

[27] Kitada, T., Asakawa, S., Hattori, N., Matsumine, H., Yamamura, Y., Minoshima, S., Yokochi, M., Mizuno, Y. and Shimizu, N., Mutations in the parkin gene cause autosomal recessive juvenile parkinsonism, *Nature*, 392 (1998) 605-8.

[28] Kogel, D., Schomburg, R., Schurmann, T., Reimertz, C., Konig, H.G., Poppe, M., Eckert, A., Muller, W.E. and Prehn, J.H., The amyloid precursor protein protects PC12 cells against endoplasmic reticulum stress-induced apoptosis, *J Neurochem*, 87 (2003) 248-56.

[29] Kondo, S., Murakami, T., Tatsumi, K., Ogata, M., Kanemoto, S., Otori, K., Iseki, K., Wanaka, A. and Imaizumi, K., OASIS, a CREB/ATF-family member, modulates UPR signalling in astrocytes, *Nat Cell Biol*, 7 (2005) 186-94.

[30] Kudo, T., Katayama, T., Imaizumi, K., Yasuda, Y., Yatera, M., Okochi, M., Tohyama, M. and Takeda, M., The unfolded protein response is involved in the pathology of Alzheimer's disease, *Ann N Y Acad Sci*, 977 (2002) 349-55.

[31] Le Bras, M., Clement, M.V., Pervaiz, S. and Brenner, C., Reactive oxygen species and the mitochondrial signaling pathway of cell death, *Histol Histopathol*, 20 (2005) 205-19.

[32] Levy-Lahad, E., Wasco, W., Poorkaj, P., Romano, D.M., Oshima, J., Pettingell, W.H., Yu, C.E., Jondro, P.D., Schmidt, S.D., Wang, K. and et al., Candidate gene for the chromosome 1 familial Alzheimer's disease locus, *Science*, 269 (1995) 973-7.

[33] Lilius, L., Froelich Fabre, S., Basun, H., Forsell, C., Axelman, K., Mattila, K., Andreadis, A., Viitanen, M., Winblad, B., Fratiglioni, L. and Lannfelt, L., Tau gene polymorphisms and apolipoprotein E epsilon4 may interact to increase risk for Alzheimer's disease, *Neurosci Lett*, 277 (1999) 29-32.

[34] Mengesdorf, T., Althausen, S., Oberndorfer, I. and Paschen, W., Response of neurons to an irreversible inhibition of endoplasmic reticulum Ca(2+)-ATPase: relationship between global protein synthesis and expression and translation of individual genes, *Biochem J*, 356 (2001) 805-12.

[35] Mori, K., Tripartite management of unfolded proteins in the endoplasmic reticulum, *Cell*, 101 (2000) 451-4.

[36] Morishima, N., Nakanishi, K., Takenouchi, H., Shibata, T. and Yasuhiko, Y., An endoplasmic reticulum stress-specific caspase cascade in apoptosis. Cytochrome c-independent activation of caspase-9 by caspase-12, *J Biol Chem*, 277 (2002) 34287-94.

[37] Morishima, N., Nakanishi, K., Tsuchiya, K., Shibata, T. and Seiwa, E., Translocation of Bim to the endoplasmic reticulum (ER) mediates ER stress signaling for activation of caspase-12 during ER stress-induced apoptosis, *J Biol Chem*, 279 (2004) 50375-81.

[38]   Nakagawa, T., Zhu, H., Morishima, N., Li, E., Xu, J., Yankner, B.A. and Yuan, J., Caspase-12 mediates endoplasmic-reticulum-specific apoptosis and cytotoxicity by amyloid-beta, *Nature*, 403 (2000) 98-103.

[39]   Nishitoh, H., Matsuzawa, A., Tobiume, K., Saegusa, K., Takeda, K., Inoue, K., Hori, S., Kakizuka, A. and Ichijo, H., ASK1 is essential for endoplasmic reticulum stress-induced neuronal cell death triggered by expanded polyglutamine repeats, *Genes Dev*, 16 (2002) 1345-55.

[40]   Oppenheim, R.W., Cell death during development of the nervous system, *Annu Rev Neurosci*, 14 (1991) 453-501.

[41]   Patapoutian, A. and Reichardt, L.F., Trk receptors: mediators of neurotrophin action, *Curr Opin Neurobiol*, 11 (2001) 272-80.

[42]   Rao, R.V. and Bredesen, D.E., Misfolded proteins, endoplasmic reticulum stress and neurodegeneration, *Curr Opin Cell Biol*, 16 (2004) 653-62.

[43]   Rao, R.V., Castro-Obregon, S., Frankowski, H., Schuler, M., Stoka, V., del Rio, G., Bredesen, D.E. and Ellerby, H.M., Coupling endoplasmic reticulum stress to the cell death program. An Apaf-1-independent intrinsic pathway, *J Biol Chem*, 277 (2002) 21836-42.

[44]   Rego, A.C. and Oliveira, C.R., Mitochondrial dysfunction and reactive oxygen species in excitotoxicity and apoptosis: implications for the pathogenesis of neurodegenerative diseases, *Neurochem Res*, 28 (2003) 1563-74.

[45]   Rubinsztein, D.C., Barton, D.E., Davison, B.C. and Ferguson-Smith, M.A., Analysis of the huntingtin gene reveals a trinucleotide-length polymorphism in the region of the gene that contains two CCG-rich stretches and a correlation between decreased age of onset of Huntington's disease and CAG repeat number, *Hum Mol Genet*, 2 (1993) 1713-5.

[46]   Schulz, J.B., Bremen, D., Reed, J.C., Lommatzsch, J., Takayama, S., Wullner, U., Loschmann, P.A., Klockgether, T. and Weller, M., Cooperative interception of neuronal apoptosis by BCL-2 and BAG-1 expression: prevention of caspase activation and reduced production of reactive oxygen species, *J Neurochem*, 69 (1997) 2075-86.

[47]   Scorrano, L., Oakes, S.A., Opferman, J.T., Cheng, E.H., Sorcinelli, M.D., Pozzan, T. and Korsmeyer, S.J., BAX and BAK regulation of endoplasmic reticulum Ca2+: a control point for apoptosis, *Science*, 300 (2003) 135-9.

[48]   Sherrington, R., Rogaev, E.I., Liang, Y., Rogaeva, E.A., Levesque, G., Ikeda, M., Chi, H., Lin, C., Li, G., Holman, K. and et al., Cloning of a gene bearing missense mutations in early-onset familial Alzheimer's disease, *Nature*, 375 (1995) 754-60.

[49]   Shimoke, K., Amano, H., Kishi, S., Uchida, H., Kudo, M. and Ikeuchi, T., Nerve growth factor attenuates endoplasmic reticulum stress-mediated apoptosis via suppression of caspase-12 activity, *J Biochem (Tokyo)*, 135 (2004) 439-46.

[50]   Shimoke, K. and Chiba, H., Nerve growth factor prevents 1-methyl-4-phenyl-1,2,3,6-tetrahydropyridine-induced cell death via the Akt pathway by suppressing caspase-3-like activity using PC12 cells: relevance to therapeutical application for Parkinson's disease, *J Neurosci Res*, 63 (2001) 402-9.

[51]   Shimoke, K., Kubo, T., Numakawa, T., Abiru, Y., Enokido, Y., Takei, N., Ikeuchi, T. and Hatanaka, H., Involvement of phosphatidylinositol-3 kinase in prevention of low K(+)-induced apoptosis of cerebellar granule neurons, *Brain Res Dev Brain Res*, 101 (1997) 197-206.

[52] Shimoke, K., Kudo, M. and Ikeuchi, T., MPTP-induced reactive oxygen species promote cell death through a gradual activation of caspase-3 without expression of GRP78/Bip as a preventive measure against ER stress in PC12 cells, *Life Sci*, 73 (2003) 581-93.

[53] Shimoke, K., Utsumi, T., Kishi, S., Nishimura, M., Sasaya, H., Kudo, M. and Ikeuchi, T., Prevention of endoplasmic reticulum stress-induced cell death by brain-derived neurotrophic factor in cultured cerebral cortical neurons, *Brain Res*, 1028 (2004) 105-11.

[54] Shimoke, K., Yamagishi, S., Yamada, M., Ikeuchi, T. and Hatanaka, H., Inhibition of phosphatidylinositol 3-kinase activity elevates c-Jun N-terminal kinase activity in apoptosis of cultured cerebellar granule neurons, *Brain Res Dev Brain Res*, 112 (1999) 245-53.

[55] Soltoff, S.P., Rabin, S.L., Cantley, L.C. and Kaplan, D.R., Nerve growth factor promotes the activation of phosphatidylinositol 3-kinase and its association with the trk tyrosine kinase, *J Biol Chem*, 267 (1992) 17472-7.

[56] Urano, F., Bertolotti, A. and Ron, D., IRE1 and efferent signaling from the endoplasmic reticulum, *J Cell Sci*, 113 Pt 21 (2000) 3697-702.

[57] Vetter, M.L., Martin-Zanca, D., Parada, L.F., Bishop, J.M. and Kaplan, D.R., Nerve growth factor rapidly stimulates tyrosine phosphorylation of phospholipase C-gamma 1 by a kinase activity associated with the product of the trk protooncogene, *Proc Natl Acad Sci U S A*, 88 (1991) 5650-4.

[58] Wang, H.G. and Reed, J.C., Mechanisms of Bcl-2 protein function, *Histol Histopathol*, 13 (1998) 521-30.

[59] Weiner, M.F., Vega, G., Risser, R.C., Honig, L.S., Cullum, C.M., Crumpacker, D. and Rosenberg, R.N., Apolipoprotein E epsilon 4, other risk factors, and course of Alzheimer's disease, *Biol Psychiatry*, 45 (1999) 633-8.

In: New Trends in Brain Research
Editor: F. J. Chen, pp. 75-94

ISBN 1-59454-834-X
© 2006 Nova Science Publishers, Inc.

Chapter IV

NEUROHYPOPHYSEAL HORMONE SECRETION DURING SEPTIC SHOCK

Maria José A. Rocha, Gabriela R. Oliveira
and Pollyanna B. Farias-Corrêa

Department of Morphology, Stomatology and Physiology. Dentistry School of Ribeirão
Preto, University of São Paulo, Ribeirão Preto, SP, Brazil

ABSTRACT

Sepsis, the systemic response to severe infection, and its complication, the septic shock, show several physiological alterations that include hypotension and changes in hormone secretion. Animal experimental models, such as LPS injection and cecal ligation and puncture can help to understand the pathophysiology of sepsis. Patterns of neurohypophyseal hormone secretion have been reported to be similar in experimental sepsis model and clinical findings. In the early phase of septic shock, elevated vasopressin plasma levels are detected; while in the late phase, these hormone levels are found to be inappropriately low, despite continuing hypotension. In order to understand why these vasopressin levels are so low, recent investigations analyzed neurohypophyseal vasopressin content and corresponding mRNA levels as indices for hormone synthesis. Further studies addressed hormone clearance, sympathetic function, the role of inflammatory mediators and neuronal activation. The neural pathways involved in hypothalamus activation during sepsis have been investigated by using c-*fos* as a marker. These studies revealed the importance of the circumventricular regions and autonomic centers in the medulla oblongata, and point to nitric oxide as the major cause for the deficiency in vasopressin secretion during the late phase of septic shock.

INTRODUCTION

Sepsis is the systemic response that results from a complex interaction between host and infectious agents. This pathophysiological process has different subsets. The first one is the systemic inflammatory response syndrome (SIRS) associated with infection and characterized by a heart rate higher than 90 beats/min, respiration more than 20 breaths/min or PCO_2 less than 32 torr, body temperature more than 38°C or less than 36°C, white blood cell counts (WBC) higher than 12.000 cells/mm^3 or less than 4.000 cells/mm^3, or more than 10% immature cells (band). This syndrome associated with hypotension (<90mmHg), organic dysfunction, perfusion abnormalities, lactic acidosis, oliguria and altered mental state is defined as severe sepsis. When the hypotension becomes refractory to adequate fluid resuscitation, the perfusion abnormalities are worsened, and the use of vasopressors are required, a patient has entered septic shock. Hypotension and hypoperfusion during septic shock can lead to a more serious stage of alteration in organ function, causing dysfunction or even total failure of organs, a syndrome denominated multiple organ dysfunction syndrome (MODS) (American College of Chest Physicians/Society of Critical Care Medicine Consensus Conference, 1992; Bone et al., 1992; Parrillo, 1993; Bone et al., 1997; Hanna, 2003).

Sepsis, septic shock and MODS are the most common causes of death in Intensive Care Units (ICU), in spite of all the technological advances. Demographic aging of the population, increased therapeutic procedures, invasive diagnoses, and the increase of immunosupression therapies are some factors that have increased the incidence of sepsis and its complications in the last decades (Bone, 1991; Parrillo, 1993; Bone et al., 1997; Angus; Wax, 2001; Hanna, 2003).

PATHOPHYSIOLOGY OF THE SEPSIS

Sepsis is a multifatorial condition with several interacting components, including genetic factors (Holmes et al., 2003; Trentzsch et al., 2003). The systemic response syndrome to infection involves inflammatory, cardiovascular and endocrine processes. The excessive response to infection results in the production of several inflammatory mediators that may cause severe functional alterations and can lead to the multiple organ dysfunction syndrome, usually accompanied by high mortality rate (Bone, 1991; Parrillo, 1993; Annane et al., 2005).

The inflammatory cascade that occurs in sepsis is generally caused by the action of bacterial cell wall components, such as lipopolysaccharide (LPS) of gram-negative bacterias, or lipoteichoic acid (LTA) of gram-positive bacterias. In addition, it may also be caused by fungi, viruses and parasites (Parrillo, 1993; Glauser et al., 1994; Sands et al., 1997; Annane et al., 2005).

Disruption of gram-negative bacteria prompts the endotoxin (LPS) release. The amount of LPS necessary to induce the inflammatory cascade and, consequently, sepsis may be quite different depending on the host (Glauser et al., 1991; Glauser et al., 1994). In the bloodstream, LPS links first to high-density lipoprotein (HDL). Then, the LPS-binding protein (LBP), a plasma protein synthesized and liberated by the liver, transfers LPS to CD14 and Toll-like receptors (TLR-4) on the surface of monocytes, macrophages and neutrophils.

Via soluble CD14, LPS also activates endotelial cells. Inflammatory mediators are rapidly produced and liberated by monocytes, macrophages, neutrophils and LPS-activated endotelial cells (Karima et al., 1999; Hanna, 2003).

Leukotriene, tumor necrosis factor (TNF), interleukin (IL)-1, IL-6, IL-8, IL-12, gamma interferon (IFN-γ), nitric oxide (NO), platelet activating factor (PAF) and prostaglandins (PGs) are some of the inflammatory mediators produced during sepsis. Many of these mediators can, on the one hand, have protecting effects, and on the other hand, can also be harmful. The complex interactions of the inflammatory mediators can be synergistic or antagonistic, increasing the response of the host to infection and limiting the inflammation, or destroying the homeostasis by stimulating the production of other mediators (Bone, 1991; Rios-Santos et al., 2003; Benjamim et al., 2005).

The excessive production of inflammatory mediators during sepsis, septic shock and MODS are, therefore, the cause for physiological alterations that include changes in the central nervous system activation and hormone secretion. In this chapter we will review the mechanisms proposed to explain neuronal activation and changes in neurohypophyseal hormone secretion that occur during clinical and experimental studies on sepsis.

MODELS OF EXPERIMENTAL SEPSIS

Several experimental models, such as intravascular infusion of endotoxin or live bacteria, bacterial peritonitis, cecal ligation and puncture (CLP), soft tissue infection, pneumonia and meningitis have been developed to study the pathophysiological aspects of sepsis (Garrido et al., 2004).

The incidence of gram-negative bacteria in sepsis cases was 45 - 60% in the past (Karima et al., 1999) and because of this fact the LPS injection model has been extensively used. The serum cytokine response to exogenous LPS injection is transient and attains a greater magnitude than can be observed clinically (Trentzsch et al., 2003). The severe hypodynamic circulatory response occurs without the initial hyperdynamic circulatory response. Another difference is that pharmacological agents and manipulation that have been shown to be effective in exogenous LPS animal models have failed in clinical trials (Fink; Heard, 1990; Riedemann et al., 2003; Overhaus et al., 2004). Although the LPS injection model has contributed to explain the activation pathways involved in the pathogenesis of sepsis, it does not represent the typical episode of clinical sepsis, but may be an adequate model of endotoxemic shock (Riedemann et al., 2003; Garrido et al., 2004; Overhaus et al., 2004).

The incidence of gram-negative sepsis has diminished over the years to 25-30% in 2000, while gram-positive and polymicrobial infections have increased to 30-50% (Martin et al., 2003; Annane et al., 2005). The mortality rate is similar to gram-positive and gram-negative bacterial infection (Hanna, 2003; Martin et al., 2003; Garrido et al., 2004). Because of this observation, other experimental models that better resemble the nowadays more frequent human bacterial infection are being used.

The cecal ligation and puncture (CLP) model is one of those models and has been used widely in sepsis research because it closely mimics clinical observations on cardiovascular and inflammatory responses induced during polymicrobial peritonitis, perforated appendicitis, diverticulitis, bacteremia and systemic sepsis (Wichterman et al., 1980; Fink; Heard, 1990;

Villa et al., 1995; Garrido et al., 2004; Overhaus et al., 2004; Westphal et al., 2004; Benjamim et al., 2005). The technical procedures are simple; the cecum is ligated distal to the ileocecal valve and punctured. The lethality of the septic stimulus can be manipulated by needle size and number of punctures (Baker et al., 1983; Garrido et al., 2004). Furthermore, it is a good animal model for sepsis in patients with colon perforation that present peritoneal contaminations with mixed microorganisms in the presence of devitalized tissue.

In the CLP model, the presence of inflammatory focus and polymicrobial infection, induces differences in the onset of endotoxemia and in the release pattern of inflammatory mediators showing a more complex response that is clearly independent of the activation of the innate immune response to LPS injection (Villa et al., 1995; Walley et al., 1996; Echtenacher et al., 2001; Trentzsch et al., 2003).

NEUROHYPOPHYSEAL HORMONES

Arginine vasopressin (AVP) and oxytocin (OT) are peptides hormones synthesized in magnocellular neurons of the supraoptic (SON) and paraventricular (PVN) nuclei of the hypothalamus and stored in the neurohypophysis (Du Vigneaud, 1954; George; Jacobowitz, 1975; Cunningham; Sawchenko, 1991). They are released into the circulation upon stimulation by increased plasma osmolality, angiotensin II, and as a reflex response to hypovolemia and hypotension (Dunn et al., 1973; George, 1976; Abboud et al., 1990; Cunningham; Sawchenko, 1991; Kadekaro et al., 1992; Windle et al., 1993; Dampney, 1994; Morris et al., 1994; Johnson; Thunhorst, 1997; Antunes-Rodrigues et al., 2004; Mckinley et al., 2004; Oliveira et al., 2004) and in fever, nausea and stress (Callahan et al., 1992; Pittman; Bagdan, 1992; Pittman; Wilkinson, 1992). Release of this hormone is also increased by endotoxins, prostaglandins and interleukin-1 (Kasting et al., 1985; Naito et al., 1991; Holmes et al., 2001; Giusti-Paiva et al., 2002; Kovacs, 2002; Mutlu; Factor, 2004; Giusti-Paiva et al., 2005).

Vasopressin is considered a weak pressor agent because it resets the cardiac baroreflex to a lower pressure by decreasing the heart rate. However, it is a more potent vasoconstrictor than angiotensin II or norepinephrine (Reid, 1997). Therefore it plays an important role in the regulation of arterial pressure. The physiological actions of AVP, summarized in Table 1, are mediated by several receptors: V1a, V1b and V2 (Cunningham; Sawchenko, 1991; Birnbaumer, 2000; Holmes et al., 2001; Mutlu; Factor, 2004; Delmas et al., 2005). In very low concentrations vasopressin may also dilatate some vascular beds, probably by stimulation of OT receptors (OTRs) and NO production in the endothelial cells (Thibonnier et al., 1999; Holmes et al., 2001; Delmas et al., 2005). Such OTRs have been found in endothelial cells of human umbilical vein, aorta, and pulmonary artery (Thibonnier et al., 1999).

Oxytocin relaxes vessels and causes a drop in mean arterial pressure, possibly through effects on the CNS, and by a mechanism that may involve a decrease in cardiac rate and force of contraction. It may also affect atrial natriuretic peptide secretion and nitric oxide production, thus contributing to the cardiovascular regulation (Gutkowska et al., 2000; Jankowski et al., 2000; Petersson, 2002).

Table 1. Vasopressin receptors and physiological effects

Receptors	Tissue	Intracellular Signaling	Principal effects
V1a receptor	Vascular smooth muscle, kidney, spleen, vesicle, testis, platelets, hepatocyte, bladder, adipocytes	Phospholipase C activation, intracellular calcium release	Vasoconstriction
V1b receptor	Hypophysis Endothelium	Via G protein, increase cAMP NO mediated	Increases ACTH secretion Vasodilatation
V2 receptor	Renal collecting duct	Via G protein, increase cAMP	Increases permeability to water
OTR	Uterus, mammary gland Endothelium	Phospholipase C activation, intracellular calcium release NO mediated	Muscle contraction Vasodilatation

ACTH, adrenocorticotrophic hormone; cAMP, cyclic adenosine monophosphate; NO, nitric oxide; OTR, oxytocin receptor.

The physiological functions of OT in the female sex are better known. Oxytocin causes uterine contractions and acts on the myoepithelial cells surrounding mammillary alveolar glands to cause milk let-down in response to suckling. It seems also to act on the smooth muscles of the vas deferens leading to ejaculation in males. Moreover, the hormone is released in response to feeding and gastric distension (Verbalis et al., 1986; Renaud et al., 1987; Cunningham; Sawchenko, 1991).

Vasopressin and oxytocin also act as neurotransmitters with effects on body temperature, behavior and blood pressure (Pittman; Bagdan, 1992; Pittman; Wilkinson, 1992; De Wied et al., 1993; Kovacs; De Wied, 1994).

NEUROHYPOPHYSEAL HORMONE DURING SEPTIC SHOCK

Vasopressin secretion in sepsis is much more studied than OT. The hormone shows a biphasic response in clinical and experimental septic shock (Landry et al., 1997; Giusti-Paiva et al., 2002; Patel et al., 2002; Delmas et al., 2005; Oliveira et al., 2005). Clinical studies report that in the initial phase of sepsis, high AVP plasma levels can be found in patients, and these may help to restore blood pressure that tends to decrease due to cytokine and NO release. However, in the late phase when the observed hypotension would normally stimulate AVP secretion, the hormone concentrations are inappropriately low, contributing to the vasodilatory shock (Landry et al., 1997; Landry; Oliver, 2001; Sharshar et al., 2003a). Vasopressin analogs have been used in patients to treat hypotension, and it was observed that the decrease in AVP level is followed by a V1-receptor hypersensitivity, which represents an advantage in the late stages of sepsis when vascular hyporesponsiveness against catecholamines complicates hemodynamic support (Landry et al., 1997; Delmas et al., 2005).

In experimental endotoxemia induced by exogenous LPS administration in rats, baboons and dogs, elevated plasma levels of AVP and OT were observed in the early period of sepsis (Wilson et al., 1981a; Wilson et al., 1981b; Kasting et al., 1985; Kasting, 1986; Giusti-Paiva et al., 2003; Giusti-Paiva et al., 2005). In the first hour after endovenous LPS injection, the plasma AVP and OT levels showed a steep increase, but in the next 6 hours, the plasma hormone levels returned to the basal level, in spite of persistent hypotension observed in some experiments (Kasting et al., 1985; Aiura et al., 1995; Andrew et al., 2000; Giusti-Paiva et al., 2002; Giusti-Paiva et al., 2005).

Westphal and colleagues (2004) also described inappropriately low AVP secretion 24 hours after CLP, when the mean arterial pressure was significantly decreased in relation to basal condition of the same animal. Recently, using different degrees of severity in the CLP experimental sepsis model in rats, we also observed a biphasic response for AVP and OT (Oliveira et al., 2005).

The reason for the inappropriately low AVP level in the late phase of septic shock is not very clear, but some mechanisms have been proposed and investigated. These include depletion of neurohypophyseal stores due to excessive secretion in the initial phase, increased vasopressinase activity, autonomic dysfunction and inhibitory effects of increased norepinephrine and nitric oxide (NO) on AVP production and/or release (Landry et al., 1997; Reid, 1997; Holmes et al., 2001; Landry; Oliver, 2001; Sharshar et al., 2002; Sharshar et al., 2003a; Brierre et al., 2004; Mutlu; Factor, 2004; Den Ouden; Meinders, 2005).

NEUROHYPOPHYSEAL STORES

Holmes and colleagues (2001) suggest that a depletion of the neurohypophyseal stocks could be one of the reasons for the diminished AVP secretion in advanced shock. In fact, depletion of AVP neurohypophyseal stores has been reported. Magnetic resonance imaging performed on septic patients with inappropriately low plasma AVP levels showed a lower signal intensity than in normal subjects, suggesting that neurohypophyseal stores of this hormone are depleted (Sharshar et al., 2002). In rats however, AVP stocks in the neurohypophysis measured 6 hours after a 1.5mg/kg LPS injection did not show any difference when compared to controls (Giusti-Paiva et al., 2002).

Analysis of mRNA levels as indices for hormone synthesis in endotoxic shock showed controversial results. In rats, a high dose of intraperitoneally injected LPS decreased AVP mRNA levels in the SON and PVN 6 hours after the stimulus (Grinevich et al., 2003). However, when LPS was administered intracisternally (200ng/kg body weight) an elevated AVP mRNA content was observed after 4 hours, but only in the SON (Boros et al., 1999). Using the sepsis model by CLP we recently analysed neurohypophyseal and hypothalamic hormone content in a time-course experiment. We found that the animals seem to be unable to restore the neurohypophyseal content in time and, thus, may not be able to supply the organism's needs during a continuous septic stimulus (data not published). Even though we could not confirm a depletion of the AVP neurohypophyseal stocks in our CLP group, there was a clear attenuated response when compared to sham animals. Whether septic shock is associated with an impaired synthesis of AVP thus remains a question still to be investigated.

VASOPRESSIN CLEARANCE AND AUTONOMIC DYSFUNCTION

Increased AVP clearance seems not to be the mechanism for the inappropriately low circulating AVP level since infusion of exogenous hormone reached the expected AVP plasma levels (Landry et al., 1997; Landry; Oliver, 2001). Moreover, circulating vasopressinase was undetectable suggesting once again that increased clearance is not an issue (Sharshar et al., 2002).

Some investigators suggest that depletion of AVP neurohypophyseal stocks may be due to intense and permanent stimulation of baroreceptors, or to a failure in the autonomous nervous system in the late phase of sepsis (Goldstein et al., 1995; Reid, 1997; Annane et al., 1999; Holmes et al., 2001; Sharshar et al., 2002). It has been proposed that high sympathetic drive may lead to saturation of low frequency oscillatory systems, or that excessive concentrations of circulating catecholamines could compromise central autonomic controls (Van De Borne et al., 1997; Annane et al., 1999). In fact, the pressor response to exogenous AVP in patients in septic shock was not associated with the expected decrease in heart rate usually observed under normal conditions (Landry et al., 1997). Additionally, high concentrations of catecholamines inhibit AVP production, and thus can contribute to the inappropriately low AVP levels in the late phase of septic shock (Day et al., 1985).

Moreover, arterial baroreflex function seems to determine the survival time in LPS-induced shock, as shown recently by Shen et al. (2004).

NITRIC OXIDE PARTICIPATION IN AVP SECRETION

Nitric oxide has been reported to participate in neurotransmission and neuroendocrine signaling in physiological and pathologic processes (Brann et al., 1997; Rivier, 2003; Kadekaro, 2004; Giusti-Paiva et al., 2005b).

It is a highly diffusible and reactive gas that has a half-life of approximately 10 seconds, and in the blood, it is rapidly metabolized to nitrite and nitrate. It can also interact with free oxygen radicals to form the oxidant peroxynitrite that may contribute to cellular toxicity. NO is generated by the enzyme nitric oxide synthase (NOS) that exists in three isoforms (Moncada et al., 1991; Thiemermann, 1997; Lamas et al., 1998; Feihl et al., 2001). The neuronal NOS (nNOS) and endothelial NOS (eNOS) are constitutively expressed and are primarily localized in neurons and endothelial cells. Their activities are regulated by changes in intracellular calcium. The inducible NOS (iNOS) is a calcium-independent isoform of the enzyme which is induced in macrophages, leukocytes, endothelial cells, smooth muscle cells, parenchymal cells and various other cell types in response to cytokines, LPS and several other inflammatory stimuli (Wang; Marsden, 1995; Moncada, 1997; Thiemermann, 1997; Lamas et al., 1998; Moncada, 1999; Feihl et al., 2001). In fact, this gas is believed to play a key role in the pathogenesis of septic shock.

The formation of NO exerts beneficial effects including vasodilatation, prevention of platelet and leukocyte adhesion, improvement of microcirculatory blood flow, and increase in host defense (Thiemermann, 1997). However, the high production of NO (iNOS-mediated) in the late phase of sepsis contributes to the deleterious effects of this syndrome, such as persistent hypotension, altered vascular permeability and organ injury (Wu et al., 1995;

Thiemermann, 1997; Titheradge, 1999; Feihl et al., 2001; Moncada; Erusalimsky, 2002; Sharshar et al., 2003b; Wu et al., 2004).

It has been suggested that NO can act centrally to modulate AVP secretion (Ota et al., 1993; Yasin et al., 1993; Giusti-Paiva et al., 2002; Ventura et al., 2002). The intracerebroventricular (i.c.v.) injection of a NO donor in conscious rats caused an increase in plasma AVP concentrations, showing a stimulatory action of NO on vasopressin release (Ota et al.,1993). However, Yasin et al (1993) observed that in the hypothalamus of intact rats, the release of AVP induced by IL-1β *in vitro* was attenuated by incubation with NO donors. This effect was reversed by non-selective NOS inhibitors. Additionally, Kadekaro (2004) showed that i.c.v. injection of NOS inhibitor (L-NAME) in conscious rats promoted an increase in plasma levels of AVP. This demonstrates that NO can have a stimulatory, as well as an inhibitory influence on AVP secretion, possibly depending on physiological context. In pathological conditions, like in endotoxemic or septic shock, the overproduction of NO in the late phase seems to be exerting an inhibitory effect in AVP release (Giusti-Paiva et al., 2002; Giusti-Paiva et al., 2003).

NOS protein and NOS mRNA have been observed in several brain areas, such as the subfornical organ (SFO), organ vasculosum of lamina terminalis (OVLT), median preoptic nucleus (MnPO), PVN, SON, and in the ventrolateral medulla (VLM) (Bredt et al., 1991; Yamada et al., 1996; Chan et al., 2001; Chan et al., 2003). Moreover, iNOS mRNA is expressed in magnocellular and parvocellular neurons in the PVN of rats injected with LPS (Harada et al., 1999).

Several investigators have suggested that NO produced in brain tissues is involved in the control of the activity of the hypothalamus-pituitary axis (Uribe et al., 1999; Giusti-Paiva et al., 2002; Rivier, 2003; Giusti-Paiva et al., 2005). Central injection of aminoguanidine (iNOS inhibitor) promoted an increase in plasma vasopressin levels and prevented blood pressure decrease in the late phase of endotoxemic shock. Intravenous inhibitor injection blocked peripheral NO production, but it was not sufficient to increase the plasma AVP concentration (Giusti-Paiva et al., 2002). In accordance with these findings, NO donors and the precursor sodium nitroprusside inhibited supraoptic vasopressin neuron activity *in vitro*, and this response was prevented by hemoglobin, a scavenger of NO. When slices of SON received a NO inhibitor, neuronal activity was enhanced (Liu et al., 1997). These results show that NO has an inhibitory influence in AVP neurons, and support the notion that centrally produced NO might modulate AVP neurons and inhibit AVP secretion in septic shock.

Moreover, there is evidence that NO might be involved in apoptosis during septic shock (Sharshar et al., 2003b; Sharshar et al., 2005). In post-mortem examinations of SON and PVN, cerebral amygdala, locus coeruleus, and medullary autonomic nuclei of 19 patients with septic shock, investigators observed neuronal and glial apoptosis in these regions (Sharshar et al., 2003b). This indicates that NO can exhibit neuronal cytotoxicity in sepsis, and this could be partly responsible for the failure of AVP release in the late phase of sepsis .

NEURAL PATHWAYS IN SEPSIS AND SEPTIC SHOCK

There is an increasing appreciation of organized interactions between the immune, autonomic and neuroendocrine systems during infection. The use of Fos-protein as a marker for neuronal activity can identify cells within neural pathways that are activated by defined stimuli (Morgan; Curran, 1991). Administration of LPS has been shown to cause intense expression of the immediate early gene (c-*fos*) in several brain regions, suggesting the participation of multiple neural circuits in the central nervous system (CNS) in response to immune challenge (Ericsson et al., 1994; Sagar et al., 1995; Konsman et al., 1999; Lin et al., 1999; Matsunaga et al., 2000; Xia; Krukoff, 2001).

Investigations have shown intense c-*fos* expression in PVN and SON following LPS injection as an endotoxemic experimental model (Sagar et al., 1995; Matsunaga et al., 2000). Although the hemodynamic responses to LPS contribute to the neuronal activation, they are not the only reason. Hypothalamic neurons are already activated by LPS, at a dose that did not alter arterial pressure (Xia; Krukoff, 2001).

As reported by other investigators (Sagar et al., 1995; Elmquist et al., 1996; Xia; Krukoff, 2001), we could see (Figure 1) that other brain regions, such as the organum vasculosum of the lamina terminalis (OVLT), the subfornical organ (SFO), and the area postrema (AP) also express c-*fos* following LPS injection These regions are highly vascularized and devoid of a blood-brain barrier, and thus are susceptible to diffusion of large molecules into the respective perivascular regions (Faraci et al., 1989; Mckinley et al., 2004). They have direct and indirect connections with the PVN and SON (Miselis, 1981; Sawchenko; Swanson, 1983; Swanson; Sawchenko, 1983; Shapiro; Miselis, 1985; Cunningham; Sawchenko, 1991; Oldfield et al., 1991; Arima et al., 1998) and may contribute to integrate information on cytokines or prostaglandins and on endocrine signals borne by circulating hormones, such as angiotensin II, all liberated during LPS administration. In septic shock, the drop in blood pressure and hypovolemia promotes a release of ANG II. This molecule has receptors in SFO, OVLT and AP and could mediate ANG II-stimulated vasopressin release (Rowe et al., 1992; Ferguson; Bains, 1996; Mckinley et al., 2004). Recently, we demonstrated that the SFO region is important for the full activation of PVN and SON neurons and for the increase in AVP and OT secretion after LPS was intravenously administered in rats. Fos immunoreactivity and AVP and OT secretion were significantly reduced when endotoxemic shock was induced by LPS in SFO lesioned rats (data not published). Lesion in the anteroventral third ventricle (AV3V), a region that encompasses the OVLT, MnPO and preoptic periventricular nucleus also reduced LPS-induced Fos immunoreactivity and AVP, OT and adrenocorticotropin (ACTH) secretion (Giusti-Paiva et al., *submitted*). These results demonstrate that the SFO and also the AV3V region can be "door-ways" for cytokines and other inflammatory mediators that are released in septic shock. In fact, all the circumventricular regions should have an important role in the signaling mechanisms in sepsis because they can function as communicating structures between the brain and the bloodstream.

Besides ANG II other mediators such as prostaglandins can be acting on the lamina terminalis and other brain areas in response to infection. There is evidence that large quantities of prostaglandin receptors, mainly EP_4 receptor, exist in OVLT and SFO, and that these are activated in systemic inflammation (Rivest et al., 2000; Zhang; Rivest, 2000).

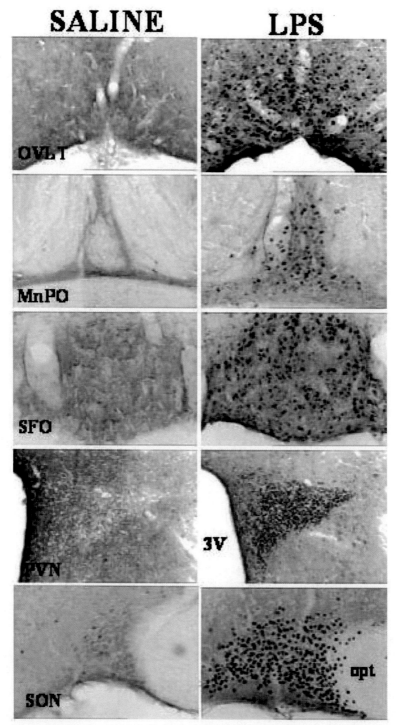

Figure 1 Neuronal activation in response to LPS or saline injection in the organ vasculosum of lamina terminalis (OVLT), median preoptic nucleus (MnPO), subfornical nucleus (SFO), paraventricular (PVN) and suproptic nuclei (SON). Abbreviations: opt, optic tract; 3V, third ventricle.

Other brain structures, like nucleus of the solitary tract (NTS), rostral ventrolateral medulla (RVLM) and caudal ventrolateral medulla (CVLM) are also activated 2 or 3 hours after intravenous LPS injection (Elmquist et al., 1996; Lin et al., 1999; Xia; Krukoff, 2001). These brain stem nuclei also have direct and indirect conections with PVN and SON (Sawchenko; Swanson, 1983; Cunningham; Sawchenko, 1991), and this indicates that they may also mediate central actions of peripherally given LPS by affecting vasopressin secretion.

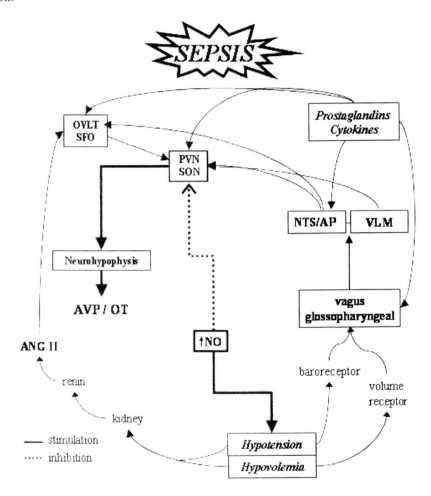

Figure 2. Schematic representation of pathways involved in neurohypophyseal hormone secretion during sepsis. Information about hypovolemia and hypotension is sensed by volume receptors and baroreceptors and conveyed via the vagus and glossopharyngeal nerve to NTS, AP and VLM. These areas project to the SON and PVN, increasing AVP and OT secretion. The brainstem areas also have input to SFO and OVLT that are activated by circulating ANG II. These nuclei have connections with PVN and SON contributing to hormone secretion. Prostaglandin and cytokines are able to directly and indirectly cause AVP and OT secretion by stimulatory effect on the nuclei involved in hormone regulation. Even though an increase in NO concentration causes hypotension that could stimulate hormone secretion, its direct effect on the SON and PVN is inhibitory.

The NTS, situated in the dorsal part of medulla oblongata, is the predominant site of termination of peripheral vagal and glossopharingeal afferents that convey information from "high pressure receptors" (or baroreceptors) and "low pressure receptors" or (volume receptors) to the central nervous system. The nucleus innervates both RVLM and CVLM regions that are involved in cardiovascular homeostasis (Cunningham; Sawchenko, 1988; Dampney, 1994). The RVLM is a site of sympathetic premotor neurons and maintains arterial pressure by providing a tonic excitation to preganglionic sympathetic neurons in the spinal cord. The CVLM has a modulatory action on RVLM neurons through a short inhibitory pathway (Ross et al., 1984; Spyer, 1990). Moreover, the NTS can receive immune-related information via the vagus nerve that senses peripheral information and conveys it to the medulla oblongata (Maier et al., 1998). Cytokines produced as a result of infections might activate vagal sensory fibers, resulting in sickness behavior and fever (Elmquist et al., 1997b). Therefore, these substrates are believed to play a role in the neuronal pathway for modulation of cardiovascular dysfunction in endotoxemic or septic shock. The brain stem nuclei therefore, can be another signaling mechanism of immune-brain interaction during septic shock that receives bloodstream information via vagus and glossopharyngeal nerves and relay it to other brain areas, such as PVN and SON (figure 2).

Central injection of prostaglandins or peripheral injection of IL-1 or LPS promoted Fos expression in the A1 cell group of the ventrolateral medulla, neurons in NTS and in PVN that express the EP_4 receptor (Zhang; Rivest, 2000). Furthermore, *in vitro* research showed that LPS-stimulated astrocytes release prostaglandin E (Fontana et al., 1982), and that rat microglia expresses prostaglandin E receptors (Caggiano; Kraig, 1999). In addition, circulating immune stimuli might activate meningeal macrophages and perivascular microglia along the borders of the brain, eliciting the local production of prostaglandins and responses, such as fever, anorexia, sleepiness, and activation of the hypothalamo-pituitary-adrenal (HPA) axis (Elmquist et al., 1997a; Elmquist et al., 1997b). Intravenous injection of LPS induces cyclooxygenase 2-like immunoreactivity in perivascular microglia along blood vessels and in meningeal macrophages at the edge of the brain (Elmquist et al., 1997a; Elmquist et al., 1997b). These studies show that prostaglandins can activate neuronal circuits in systemic inflammation and can influence pituitary hormone secretion.

All this evidence supports the idea that there is a participation of a variety of brain neural systems in endotoxemia to maintain cardiovascular and endocrine regulation. The neuronal activation can reflect the changes in vasopressin, oxytocin and adrenocorticotropin secretion during sepsis. In fact, we recently saw a decrease in c-*fos* expression in the late phase of sepsis induced by CLP in accordance with the impaired vasopressin secretion observed in this constellation (data not published).

CONCLUSION

In septic shock, inappropriately low plasma levels of vasopressin seem to be related to a depletion of vasopressin stores in the neurohypophysis. This is probably due to permanent stimulation of baroreceptors, caused by the progressively decrease of blood pressure as a consequence of overproduction of NO. Moreover, high levels of NO and catecholamines may act directly on the hypothalamic nuclei causing an inhibiton in synthesis and/or release of vasopressin.

ACKNOWLEDGEMENTS

We thank Beatriz de Carvalho-Borges for providing the immunocytochemistry results of figure 1 and Klaus Hartfelder for correcting the English. Financial support by FAPESP.

REFERENCE

Abboud, F.M., Floras, J.S., Aylward, P.E., Guo, G.B., Gupta, B.N., Schmid, P.G. Role of vasopressin in cardiovascular and blood pressure regulation. *Blood Vessels*, 1990, 27, 106-115.

Aiura, K., Ueda, M., Endo, M., Kitajima, M. Circulating concentrations and physiologic role of atrial natriuretic peptide during endotoxic shock in the rat. *Crit Care Med*, 1995, 23, 1898-1906.

American College of Chest Physicians/Society of Critical Care Medicine Consensus Conference: definitions for sepsis and organ failure and guidelines for the use of innovative therapies in sepsis. *Crit Care Med*, 1992, 20, 864-874.

Andrew, P., Deng, Y., Kaufman, S. Fluid extravasation from spleen reduces blood volume in endotoxemia. *Am J Physiol Regul Integr Comp Physiol*, 2000, 278, R60-65.

Angus, D.C., Wax, R.S. Epidemiology of sepsis: an update. *Crit Care Med*, 2001, 29, S109-116.

Annane, D., Trabold, F., Sharshar, T., Jarrin, I., Blanc, A.S., Raphael, J.C., Gajdos, P. Inappropriate sympathetic activation at onset of septic shock: a spectral analysis approach. *Am J Respir Crit Care Med*, 1999, 160, 458-465.

Annane, D., Bellissant, E., Cavaillon, J.M. Septic shock. *Lancet*, 2005, 365, 63-78.

Antunes-Rodrigues, J., De Castro, M., Elias, L.L., Valenca, M.M., Mccann, S.M. Neuroendocrine control of body fluid metabolism. *Physiol Rev*, 2004, 84, 169-208.

Arima, H., Kondo, K., Murase, T., Yokoi, H., Iwasaki, Y., Saito, H., Oiso, Y. Regulation of vasopressin synthesis and release by area postrema in rats. *Endocrinology*, 1998, 139, 1481-1486.

Baker, C.C., Chaudry, I.H., Gaines, H.O., Baue, A.E. Evaluation of factors affecting mortality rate after sepsis in a murine cecal ligation and puncture model. *Surgery*, 1983, 94, 331-335.

Benjamim, C.F., Canetti, C., Cunha, F.Q., Kunkel, S.L., Peters-Golden, M. Opposing and Hierarchical Roles of Leukotrienes in Local Innate Immune versus Vascular Responses in a Model of Sepsis. *J Immunol*, 2005, 174, 1616-1620.

Birnbaumer, M. Vasopressin receptors. *Trends Endocrinol Metab*, 2000, 11, 406-410.

Bone, R.C. The pathogenesis of sepsis. *Ann Intern Med*, 1991, 115, 457-469.

Bone, R.C., Sibbald, W.J., Sprung, C.L. The ACCP-SCCM consensus conference on sepsis and organ failure. *Chest*, 1992, 101, 1481-1483.

Bone, R.C., Grodzin, C.J., Balk, R.A. Sepsis: a new hypothesis for pathogenesis of the disease process. *Chest*, 1997, 112, 235-243.

Boros, A., Temesvari, P., Szoke, L., Vecsernyes, M., Bari, F., Abraham, C.S., Pinter, S., Gulya, K. Differential regulation of vasopressin gene expression in the hypothalamus of endotoxin-treated 14-day-old rat. *Life Sci*, 1999, 65, PL47-52.

Brann, D.W., Bhat, G.K., Lamar, C.A., Mahesh, V.B. Gaseous transmitters and neuroendocrine regulation. *Neuroendocrinology*, 1997, 65, 385-395.

Bredt, D.S., Glatt, C.E., Hwang, P.M., Fotuhi, M., Dawson, T.M., Snyder, S.H. Nitric oxide synthase protein and mRNA are discretely localized in neuronal populations of the mammalian CNS together with NADPH diaphorase. *Neuron*, 1991, 7, 615-624.

Brierre, S., Kumari, R., Deboisblanc, B.P. The endocrine system during sepsis. *Am J Med Sci*, 2004, 328, 238-247.

Caggiano, A.O., Kraig, R.P. Prostaglandin E receptor subtypes in cultured rat microglia and their role in reducing lipopolysaccharide-induced interleukin-1beta production. *J Neurochem*, 1999, 72, 565-575.

Callahan, M.F., Da Rocha, M.J., Morris, M. Sinoaortic denervation does not increase cardiovascular/endocrine responses to stress. *Neuroendocrinology*, 1992, 56, 735-744.

Chan, J.Y., Wang, S.H., Chan, S.H. Differential roles of iNOS and nNOS at rostral ventrolateral medulla during experimental endotoxemia in the rat. *Shock*, 2001, 15, 65-72.

Chan, J.Y., Wang, L.L., Ou, C.C., Chan, S.H. Downregulation of angiotensin subtype 1 receptor in rostral ventrolateral medulla during endotoxemia. *Hypertension*, 2003, 42, 103-109.

Cunningham, E.T., Jr., Sawchenko, P.E. Anatomical specificity of noradrenergic inputs to the paraventricular and supraoptic nuclei of the rat hypothalamus. *J Comp Neurol*, 1988, 274, 60-76.

Cunningham, E.T., Jr., Sawchenko, P.E. Reflex control of magnocellular vasopressin and oxytocin secretion. *Trends Neurosci*, 1991, 14, 406-411.

Dampney, R.A. Functional organization of central pathways regulating the cardiovascular system. *Physiol Rev*, 1994, 74, 323-364.

Day, T.A., Randle, J.C., Renaud, L.P. Opposing alpha- and beta-adrenergic mechanisms mediate dose-dependent actions of noradrenaline on supraoptic vasopressin neurones in vivo. *Brain Res*, 1985, 358, 171-179.

De Wied, D., Diamant, M., Fodor, M. Central nervous system effects of the neurohypophyseal hormones and related peptides. *Front Neuroendocrinol*, 1993, 14, 251-302.

Delmas, A., Leone, M., Rousseau, S., Albanese, J., Martin, C. Clinical review: Vasopressin and terlipressin in septic shock patients. *Crit Care*, 2005, 9, 212-222.

Den Ouden, D.T., Meinders, A.E. Vasopressin: physiology and clinical use in patients with vasodilatory shock: a review. *Neth J Med*, 2005, 63, 4-13.

Du Vigneaud, V. Hormones of the posterior pituitary gland: oxytocin and vasopressin. *Harvey Lect*, 1954, 50, 1-26.

Dunn, F.L., Brennan, T.J., Nelson, A.E., Robertson, G.L. The role of blood osmolality and volume in regulating vasopressin secretion in the rat. *J Clin Invest*, 1973, 52, 3212-3219.

Echtenacher, B., Freudenberg, M.A., Jack, R.S., Mannel, D.N. Differences in innate defense mechanisms in endotoxemia and polymicrobial septic peritonitis. *Infect Immun*, 2001, 69, 7271-7276.

Elmquist, J.K., Scammell, T.E., Jacobson, C.D., Saper, C.B. Distribution of Fos-like immunoreactivity in the rat brain following intravenous lipopolysaccharide administration. *J Comp Neurol*, 1996, 371, 85-103.

Elmquist, J.K., Breder, C.D., Sherin, J.E., Scammell, T.E., Hickey, W.F., Dewitt, D., Saper, C.B. Intravenous lipopolysaccharide induces cyclooxygenase 2-like immunoreactivity in rat brain perivascular microglia and meningeal macrophages. *J Comp Neurol*, 1997a, 381, 119-129.

Elmquist, J.K., Scammell, T.E., Saper, C.B. Mechanisms of CNS response to systemic immune challenge: the febrile response. *Trends Neurosci*, 1997b, 20, 565-570.

Ericsson, A., Kovacs, K.J., Sawchenko, P.E. A functional anatomical analysis of central pathways subserving the effects of interleukin-1 on stress-related neuroendocrine neurons. *J Neurosci*, 1994, 14, 897-913.

Faraci, F.M., Choi, J., Baumbach, G.L., Mayhan, W.G., Heistad, D.D. Microcirculation of the area postrema. Permeability and vascular responses. *Circ Res*, 1989, 65, 417-425.

Feihl, F., Waeber, B., Liaudet, L. Is nitric oxide overproduction the target of choice for the management of septic shock? *Pharmacol Ther*, 2001, 91, 179-213.

Ferguson, A.V., Bains, J.S. Electrophysiology of the circumventricular organs. *Front Neuroendocrinol*, 1996, 17, 440-475.

Fink, M.P., Heard, S.O. Laboratory models of sepsis and septic shock. *J Surg Res*, 1990, 49, 186-196.

Fontana, A., Kristensen, F., Dubs, R., Gemsa, D., Weber, E. Production of prostaglandin E and an interleukin-1 like factor by cultured astrocytes and C6 glioma cells. *J Immunol*, 1982, 129, 2413-2419.

Garrido, A.J., Poli De Figueiredo, L.F., Rocha E Silva, M. Experimental models of sepsis and septic shock: an overview. *Acta Cir Bras*, 2004, 19, 82-88.

George, J.M., Jacobowitz, D.M. Localization of vasopressin in discrete areas of the rat hypothalamus. *Brain Res*, 1975, 93, 363-366.

George, J.M. Vasopressin and oxytocin are depleted from rat hypothalamic nuclei after oral hypertonic saline. *Science*, 1976, 193, 146-148.

Giusti-Paiva, A., De Castro, M., Antunes-Rodrigues, J., Carnio, E.C. Inducible nitric oxide synthase pathway in the central nervous system and vasopressin release during experimental septic shock. *Crit Care Med*, 2002, 30, 1306-1310.

Giusti-Paiva, A., Ruginsk, S.G., De Castro, M., Elias, L.L., Carnio, E.C., Antunes-Rodrigues, J. Role of nitric oxide in lipopolysaccharide-induced release of vasopressin in rats. *Neurosci Lett*, 2003, 346, 21-24.

Giusti-Paiva, A., Elias, L.L., Antunes-Rodrigues, J. Inhibitory effect of gaseous neuromodulators in vasopressin and oxytocin release induced by endotoxin in rats. *Neurosci Lett*, 2005, 381, 320-324.

Giusti-Paiva, A., Carvalho-Borges, B., Carnio, E.C., Elias, L.L.K., Antunes-Rodrigues, J., Rocha, M.J.A. Lesion of the anteroventral third ventricle reduces hypothalamic activation and hypophyseal hormone secretion induced by lipopolysaccharide in rats. *Submitted*.

Glauser, M.P., Zanetti, G., Baumgartner, J.D., Cohen, J. Septic shock: pathogenesis. *Lancet*, 1991, 338, 732-736.

Glauser, M.P., Heumann, D., Baumgartner, J.D., Cohen, J. Pathogenesis and potential strategies for prevention and treatment of septic shock: an update. *Clin Infect Dis*, 1994, 18 Suppl 2, S205-216.

Goldstein, B., Kempski, M.H., Stair, D., Tipton, R.B., Deking, D., Delong, D.J., Deasla, R., Cox, C., Lund, N., Woolf, P.D. Autonomic modulation of heart rate variability during endotoxin shock in rabbits. *Crit Care Med*, 1995, 23, 1694-1702.

Grinevich, V., Ma, X.M., Jirikowski, G., Verbalis, J., Aguilera, G. Lipopolysaccharide endotoxin potentiates the effect of osmotic stimulation on vasopressin synthesis and secretion in the rat hypothalamus. *J Neuroendocrinol*, 2003, 15, 141-149.

Gutkowska, J., Jankowski, M., Mukaddam-Daher, S., Mccann, S.M. Oxytocin is a cardiovascular hormone. *Braz J Med Biol Res*, 2000, 33, 625-633.

Hanna, N. Sepsis and septic shock. *Topics in Emergency Medicine*, 2003, 25, 158-165.

Harada, S., Imaki, T., Chikada, N., Naruse, M., Demura, H. Distinct distribution and time-course changes in neuronal nitric oxide synthase and inducible NOS in the paraventricular nucleus following lipopolysaccharide injection. *Brain Res*, 1999, 821, 322-332.

Holmes, C.L., Patel, B.M., Russell, J.A., Walley, K.R. Physiology of vasopressin relevant to management of septic shock. *Chest*, 2001, 120, 989-1002.

Holmes, C.L., Russell, J.A., Walley, K.R. Genetic polymorphisms in sepsis and septic shock: role in prognosis and potential for therapy. *Chest*, 2003, 124, 1103-1115.

Jankowski, M., Wang, D., Hajjar, F., Mukaddam-Daher, S., Mccann, S.M., Gutkowska, J. Oxytocin and its receptors are synthesized in the rat vasculature. *Proc Natl Acad Sci U S A*, 2000, 97, 6207-6211.

Johnson, A.K., Thunhorst, R.L. The neuroendocrinology of thirst and salt appetite: visceral sensory signals and mechanisms of central integration. *Front Neuroendocrinol*, 1997, 18, 292-353.

Kadekaro, M., Summy-Long, J.Y., Freeman, S., Harris, J.S., Terrell, M.L., Eisenberg, H.M. Cerebral metabolic responses and vasopressin and oxytocin secretions during progressive water deprivation in rats. *Am J Physiol*, 1992, 262, R310-317.

Kadekaro, M. Nitric oxide modulation of the hypothalamo-neurohypophyseal system. *Braz J Med Biol Res*, 2004, 37, 441-450.

Karima, R., Matsumoto, S., Higashi, H., Matsushima, K. The molecular pathogenesis of endotoxic shock and organ failure. *Mol Med Today*, 1999, 5, 123-132.

Kasting, N.W., Mazurek, M.F., Martin, J.B. Endotoxin increases vasopressin release independently of known physiological stimuli. *Am J Physiol*, 1985, 248, E420-424.

Kasting, N.W. Characteristics of body temperature, vasopressin, and oxytocin responses to endotoxin in the rat. *Can J Physiol Pharmacol*, 1986, 64, 1575-1578.

Konsman, J.P., Kelley, K., Dantzer, R. Temporal and spatial relationships between lipopolysaccharide-induced expression of Fos, interleukin-1beta and inducible nitric oxide synthase in rat brain. *Neuroscience*, 1999, 89, 535-548.

Kovacs, G.L., De Wied, D. Peptidergic modulation of learning and memory processes. *Pharmacol Rev*, 1994, 46, 269-291.

Kovacs, K.J. Neurohypophyseal hormones in the integration of physiological responses to immune challenges. *Prog Brain Res*, 2002, 139, 127-146.

Lamas, S., Perez-Sala, D., Moncada, S. Nitric oxide: from discovery to the clinic. *Trends Pharmacol Sci*, 1998, 19, 436-438.

Landry, D.W., Levin, H.R., Gallant, E.M., Ashton, R.C., Jr., Seo, S., D'alessandro, D., Oz, M.C., Oliver, J.A. Vasopressin deficiency contributes to the vasodilation of septic shock. *Circulation*, 1997, 95, 1122-1125.

Landry, D.W., Oliver, J.A. The pathogenesis of vasodilatory shock. *N Engl J Med*, 2001, 345, 588-595.

Lin, H.C., Wan, F.J., Kang, B.H., Wu, C.C., Tseng, C.J. Systemic administration of lipopolysaccharide induces release of nitric oxide and glutamate and c-fos expression in the nucleus tractus solitarii of rats. *Hypertension*, 1999, 33, 1218-1224.

Liu, Q.S., Jia, Y.S., Ju, G. Nitric oxide inhibits neuronal activity in the supraoptic nucleus of the rat hypothalamic slices. *Brain Res Bull*, 1997, 43, 121-125.

Maier, S.F., Goehler, L.E., Fleshner, M., Watkins, L.R. The role of the vagus nerve in cytokine-to-brain communication. *Ann N Y Acad Sci*, 1998, 840, 289-300.

Martin, G.S., Mannino, D.M., Eaton, S., Moss, M. The epidemiology of sepsis in the United States from 1979 through 2000. *N Engl J Med*, 2003, 348, 1546-1554.

Matsunaga, W., Miyata, S., Takamata, A., Bun, H., Nakashima, T., Kiyohara, T. LPS-induced Fos expression in oxytocin and vasopressin neurons of the rat hypothalamus. *Brain Res*, 2000, 858, 9-18.

Mckinley, M.J., Mathai, M.L., Mcallen, R.M., Mcclear, R.C., Miselis, R.R., Pennington, G.L., Vivas, L., Wade, J.D., Oldfield, B.J. Vasopressin secretion: osmotic and hormonal regulation by the lamina terminalis. *J Neuroendocrinol*, 2004, 16, 340-347.

Miselis, R.R. The efferent projections of the subfornical organ of the rat: a circumventricular organ within a neural network subserving water balance. *Brain Res*, 1981, 230, 1-23.

Moncada, S., Palmer, R.M., Higgs, E.A. Nitric oxide: physiology, pathophysiology, and pharmacology. *Pharmacol Rev*, 1991, 43, 109-142.

Moncada, S. Nitric oxide in the vasculature: physiology and pathophysiology. *Ann N Y Acad Sci*, 1997, 811, 60-67; discussion 67-69.

Moncada, S. Nitric oxide: discovery and impact on clinical medicine. *J R Soc Med*, 1999, 92, 164-169.

Moncada, S., Erusalimsky, J.D. Does nitric oxide modulate mitochondrial energy generation and apoptosis? *Nat Rev Mol Cell Biol*, 2002, 3, 214-220.

Morgan, J.I., Curran, T. Stimulus-transcription coupling in the nervous system: involvement of the inducible proto-oncogenes fos and jun. *Annu Rev Neurosci*, 1991, 14, 421-451.

Morris, M., Rocha, M.J., Sim, L.J., Johnson, A.K., Callahan, M.F. Dissociation between vasopressin and oxytocin mRNA and peptide secretion after AV3V lesions. *Am J Physiol*, 1994, 267, R1640-1645.

Mutlu, G M., Factor, P. Role of vasopressin in the management of septic shock. *Intensive Care Med*, 2004, 30, 1276-1291.

Naito, Y., Fukata, J., Shindo, K., Ebisui, O., Murakami, N., Tominaga, T., Nakai, Y., Mori, K., Kasting, N.W., Imura, H. Effects of interleukins on plasma arginine vasopressin and oxytocin levels in conscious, freely moving rats. *Biochem Biophys Res Commun*, 1991, 174, 1189-1195.

Oldfield, B.J., Miselis, R.R., Mckinley, M.J. Median preoptic nucleus projections to vasopressin-containing neurones of the supraoptic nucleus in sheep. A light and electron microscopic study. *Brain Res*, 1991, 542, 193-200.

Oliveira, G.R., Franci, C.R., Rodovalho, G.V., Franci, J.A., Morris, M., Rocha, M.J. Alterations in the central vasopressin and oxytocin axis after lesion of a brain osmotic sensory region. *Brain Res Bull*, 2004, 63, 515-520.

Oliveira, G.R., Elias, L.L.K., Antunes-Rodrigues, J., Rocha, M.J.A. Time course of nitric oxide formation and secretion of vasopressin and oxytocin in an experimental model of polymicrobial sepsis. *The FASEB Journal, a multidisciplinary resource for the life sciences (Abstract)*, 2005, 19, A1222.

Ota, M., Crofton, J.T., Festavan, G.T., Share, L. Evidence that nitric oxide can act centrally to stimulate vasopressin release. *Neuroendocrinology*, 1993, 57, 955-959.

Overhaus, M., Togel, S., Pezzone, M.A., Bauer, A.J. Mechanisms of polymicrobial sepsis-induced ileus. *Am J Physiol Gastrointest Liver Physiol*, 2004, 287, G685-694.

Parrillo, J.E. Pathogenetic mechanisms of septic shock. *N Engl J Med*, 1993, 328, 1471-1477.

Patel, B.M., Chittock, D.R., Russell, J.A., Walley, K.R. Beneficial effects of short-term vasopressin infusion during severe septic shock. *Anesthesiology*, 2002, 96, 576-582.

Petersson, M. Cardiovascular effects of oxytocin. *Prog Brain Res*, 2002, 139, 281-288.

Pittman, Q.J., Bagdan, B. Vasopressin involvement in central control of blood pressure. *Prog Brain Res*, 1992, 91, 69-74.

Pittman, Q.J., Wilkinson, M.F. Central arginine vasopressin and endogenous antipyresis. *Can J Physiol Pharmacol*, 1992, 70, 786-790.

Reid, I.A. Role of vasopressin deficiency in the vasodilation of septic shock. *Circulation*, 1997, 95, 1108-1110.

Renaud, L.P., Tang, M., Mccann, M.J., Stricker, E.M., Verbalis, J.G. Cholecystokinin and gastric distension activate oxytocinergic cells in rat hypothalamus. *Am J Physiol*, 1987, 253, R661-665.

Riedemann, N.C., Guo, R.F., Ward, P.A. The enigma of sepsis. *J Clin Invest*, 2003, 112, 460-467.

Rios-Santos, F., Benjamim, C.F., Zavery, D., Ferreira, S.H., Cunha Fde, Q. A critical role of leukotriene B4 in neutrophil migration to infectious focus in cecal ligaton and puncture sepsis. *Shock*, 2003, 19, 61-65.

Rivest, S., Lacroix, S., Vallieres, L., Nadeau, S., Zhang, J., Laflamme, N. How the blood talks to the brain parenchyma and the paraventricular nucleus of the hypothalamus during systemic inflammatory and infectious stimuli. *Proc Soc Exp Biol Med*, 2000, 223, 22-38.

Rivier, C. Role of nitric oxide in regulating the rat hypothalamic-pituitary-adrenal axis response to endotoxemia. *Ann N Y Acad Sci*, 2003, 992, 72-85.

Ross, C.A., Ruggiero, D.A., Park, D.H., Joh, T.H., Sved, A.F., Fernandez-Pardal, J., Saavedra, J.M., Reis, D.J. Tonic vasomotor control by the rostral ventrolateral medulla: effect of electrical or chemical stimulation of the area containing C1 adrenaline neurons on arterial pressure, heart rate, and plasma catecholamines and vasopressin. *J Neurosci*, 1984, 4, 474-494.

Rowe, B.P., Saylor, D.L., Speth, R.C. Analysis of angiotensin II receptor subtypes in individual rat brain nuclei. *Neuroendocrinology*, 1992, 55, 563-573.

Sagar, S.M., Price, K.J., Kasting, N.W., Sharp, F.R. Anatomic patterns of Fos immunostaining in rat brain following systemic endotoxin administration. *Brain Res Bull*, 1995, 36, 381-392.

Sands, K.E., Bates, D.W., Lanken, P.N., Graman, P.S., Hibberd, P.L., Kahn, K.L., Parsonnet, J., Panzer, R., Orav, E.J., Snydman, D.R. Epidemiology of sepsis syndrome in 8 academic medical centers. Academic Medical Center Consortium Sepsis Project Working Group. *Jama*, 1997, 278, 234-240.

Sawchenko, P.E., Swanson, L.W. The organization and biochemical specificity of afferent projections to the paraventricular and supraoptic nuclei. *Prog Brain Res*, 1983, 60, 19-29.

Shapiro, R.E., Miselis, R.R. The central neural connections of the area postrema of the rat. *J Comp Neurol*, 1985, 234, 344-364.

Sharshar, T., Carlier, R., Blanchard, A., Feydy, A., Gray, F., Paillard, M., Raphael, J.C., Gajdos, P., Annane, D. Depletion of neurohypophyseal content of vasopressin in septic shock. *Crit Care Med*, 2002, 30, 497-500.

Sharshar, T., Blanchard, A., Paillard, M., Raphael, J.C., Gajdos, P., Annane, D. Circulating vasopressin levels in septic shock. *Crit Care Med*, 2003a, 31, 1752-1758.

Sharshar, T., Gray, F., Lorin De La Grandmaison, G., Hopkinson, N.S., Ross, E., Dorandeu, A., Orlikowski, D., Raphael, J.C., Gajdos, P., Annane, D. Apoptosis of neurons in cardiovascular autonomic centres triggered by inducible nitric oxide synthase after death from septic shock. *Lancet*, 2003b, 362, 1799-1805.

Sharshar, T., Hopkinson, N.S., Orlikowski, D., Annane, D. Science review: The brain in sepsis--culprit and victim. *Crit Care*, 2005, 9, 37-44.

Shen, F.M., Guan, Y.F., Xie, H.H., Su, D.F. Arterial baroreflex function determines the survival time in lipopolysaccharide-induced shock in rats. *Shock*, 2004, 21, 556-560.

Spyer, K.M. The central nervous organization of reflex circulatory control. In: Spyer, K. M., Spyer, K. M. *Central regulation of autonomic functions*, New York: Oxford University Press, 1990, 168-188.

Swanson, L.W., Sawchenko, P.E. Hypothalamic integration: organization of the paraventricular and supraoptic nuclei. *Annu Rev Neurosci*, 1983, 6, 269-324.

Thibonnier, M., Conarty, D.M., Preston, J.A., Plesnicher, C.L., Dweik, R.A., Erzurum, S.C. Human vascular endothelial cells express oxytocin receptors. *Endocrinology*, 1999, 140, 1301-1309.

Thiemermann, C. Nitric oxide and septic shock. *Gen Pharmacol*, 1997, 29, 159-166.

Titheradge, M.A. Nitric oxide in septic shock. *Biochim Biophys Acta*, 1999, 1411, 437-455.

Trentzsch, H., Stewart, D., Paidas, C.N., De Maio, A. The combination of polymicrobial sepsis and endotoxin results in an inflammatory process that could not be predicted from the independent insults. *J Surg Res*, 2003, 111, 203-208.

Uribe, R.M., Lee, S., Rivier, C. Endotoxin stimulates nitric oxide production in the paraventricular nucleus of the hypothalamus through nitric oxide synthase I: correlation with hypothalamic-pituitary-adrenal axis activation. *Endocrinology*, 1999, 140, 5971-5981.

Van De Borne, P., Montano, N., Pagani, M., Oren, R., Somers, V.K. Absence of low-frequency variability of sympathetic nerve activity in severe heart failure. *Circulation*, 1997, 95, 1449-1454.

Ventura, R.R., Gomes, D.A., Reis, W.L., Elias, L.L., Castro, M., Valenca, M.M., Carnio, E.C., Rettori, V., Mccann, S.M., Antunes-Rodrigues, J. Nitrergic modulation of vasopressin, oxytocin and atrial natriuretic peptide secretion in response to sodium intake and hypertonic blood volume expansion. *Braz J Med Biol Res*, 2002, 35, 1101-1109.

Verbalis, J.G., Mccann, M.J., Mchale, C.M., Stricker, E.M. Oxytocin secretion in response to cholecystokinin and food: differentiation of nausea from satiety. *Science*, 1986, 232, 1417-1419.

Villa, P., Sartor, G., Angelini, M., Sironi, M., Conni, M., Gnocchi, P., Isetta, A.M., Grau, G., Buurman, W., Van Tits, L.J., Et Al. Pattern of cytokines and pharmacomodulation in sepsis induced by cecal ligation and puncture compared with that induced by endotoxin. *Clin Diagn Lab Immunol*, 1995, 2, 549-553.

Walley, K.R., Lukacs, N.W., Standiford, T.J., Strieter, R.M., Kunkel, S.L. Balance of inflammatory cytokines related to severity and mortality of murine sepsis. *Infect Immun*, 1996, 64, 4733-4738.

Wang, Y., Marsden, P.A. Nitric oxide synthases: biochemical and molecular regulation. *Curr Opin Nephrol Hypertens*, 1995, 4, 12-22.

Westphal, M., Freise, H., Kehrel, B.E., Bone, H.G., Van Aken, H., Sielenkamper, A.W. Arginine vasopressin compromises gut mucosal microcirculation in septic rats. *Crit Care Med*, 2004, 32, 194-200.

Wichterman, K.A., Baue, A.E., Chaudry, I.H. Sepsis and septic shock--a review of laboratory models and a proposal. *J Surg Res*, 1980, 29, 189-201.

Wilson, M.F., Brackett, D.J., Hinshaw, L.B., Tompkins, P., Archer, L.T., Benjamin, B.A. Vasopressin release during sepsis and septic shock in baboons and dogs. *Surg Gynecol Obstet*, 1981a, 153, 869-872.

Wilson, M.F., Brackett, D.J., Tompkins, P., Benjamin, B., Archer, L.T., Hinshaw, L.B. Elevated plasma vasopressin concentrations during endotoxin and E. coli shock. *Adv Shock Res*, 1981b, 6, 15-26.

Windle, R.J., Forsling, M.L., Smith, C.P., Balment, R.J. Patterns of neurohypophysial hormone release during dehydration in the rat. *J Endocrinol*, 1993, 137, 311-319.

Wu, C.C., Chen, S.J., Szabo, C., Thiemermann, C., Vane, J.R. Aminoguanidine attenuates the delayed circulatory failure and improves survival in rodent models of endotoxic shock. *Br J Pharmacol*, 1995, 114, 1666-1672.

Wu, F., Wilson, J.X., Tyml, K. Ascorbate protects against impaired arteriolar constriction in sepsis by inhibiting inducible nitric oxide synthase expression. *Free Radic Biol Med*, 2004, 37, 1282-1289.

Xia, Y., Krukoff, T.L. Cardiovascular responses to subseptic doses of endotoxin contribute to differential neuronal activation in rat brain. *Brain Res Mol Brain Res*, 2001, 89, 71-85.

Yamada, K., Emson, P., Hokfelt, T. Immunohistochemical mapping of nitric oxide synthase in the rat hypothalamus and colocalization with neuropeptides. *J Chem Neuroanat*, 1996, 10, 295-316.

Yasin, S., Costa, A., Trainer, P., Windle, R., Forsling, M.L., Grossman, A. Nitric oxide modulates the release of vasopressin from rat hypothalamic explants. *Endocrinology*, 1993, 133, 1466-1469.

Zhang, J., Rivest, S. A functional analysis of EP4 receptor-expressing neurons in mediating the action of prostaglandin E2 within specific nuclei of the brain in response to circulating interleukin-1beta. *J Neurochem*, 2000, 74, 2134-2145.

In: New Trends in Brain Research
Editor: F. J. Chen, pp. 95-126

ISBN 1-59454-834-X
© 2006 Nova Science Publishers, Inc.

Chapter V

ROLE OF CENTRAL α_2-ADRENERGIC/IMIDAZOLINE RECEPTORS IN THE CONTROL OF THIRST, SODIUM APPETITE AND RENAL EXCRETION

José V. Menani, Lisandra B. de Oliveira, Carina A. F. de Andrade,
Alexandre M. Sugawara and Laurival A. De Luca Jr.*
Department of Physiology and Pathology, School of Dentistry, Paulista State University,
UNESP, Araraquara, SP, Brazil

ABSTRACT

Activation of central α_2-adrenergic/imidazoline receptors produces several responses that counteract increases in arterial pressure and volume expansion. The α_2-adrenergic/imidazoline agonists like clonidine and moxonidine acting centrally inhibit sympathetic activity, thirst and sodium appetite and induce diuresis and natriuresis. The involvement of central α_2-adrenergic vs. imidazoline receptors has been subjected to controversies, but there is also evidence that both receptors may interact in some of these responses. A stronger inhibitory effect on thirst and sodium appetite is produced by mixed α_2-adrenergic/imidazoline agonists, than by selective α_2-adrenergic agonists; an effect likely independent from activation of presynaptic α_2-adrenergic receptors. Mixed α_2-adrenergic/imidazoline antagonists are also much more potent than non-imidazoline antagonists to inhibit the agonists. Although the anti-hypertensive effects of α_2-adrenergic/imidazoline agonists is dependent on hindbrain areas, injections of the α_2-adrenergic/imidazoline agonists inhibit water intake and induces diuresis and natriuresis when injected into the lateral ventricle (LV), but not into the 4th ventricle (4th V). On the

---

* *Correspondence*: José Vanderlei Menani, Ph.D. Dept. of Physiology and Pathology, School of Dentistry, UNESP; Rua Humaitá 1680, 14801-903, Araraquara, SP, Brazil. Phone: +55 (16) 3301-6486; FAX: +55 (16) 3301-6488; E-mail: menani@foar.unesp.br

other hand inhibition of sodium appetite is produced by injections of α_2-adrenergic/imidazoline agonists into the LV or 4th V. In spite of the established inhibitory effect of centrally acting α_2-adrenergic/imidazoline agonists on water and NaCl intake, recent results from our laboratory have shown that injections of moxonidine or clonidine into the lateral parabrachial nucleus (LPBN) strongly increase hypertonic NaCl intake and abolish the effects of the activation of the inhibitory LPBN serotonergic mechanisms. Therefore, the central activation of α_2-adrenergic/imidazoline receptors through the ventricular system inhibits sodium intake, but activation of the same type of receptors in the LPBN strongly increases sodium intake probably by the blockade of the serotonergic inhibitory mechanisms.

Keywords: α_2-adrenoceptors, behavior, water intake, sodium intake, natriuresis, diuresis.

INTRODUCTION

Functional studies on the role of central neurotransmitters in behavior, particularly in the rat, were mostly improved by techniques that allow the delivery of chemicals directly into the central nervous system. Noradrenaline was one of those chemicals tested in early works of intrahypothalamic injections leading to induction of feeding and inhibition of drinking [Grossman, 1962]. Later works have shown that the function of central noradrenaline in the control of fluid intake does not follow a simple rule and it depends on the area of the encephalon studied, the type of treatment the animal receives and the receptor involved. Alpha$_1$ and β- adrenergic receptors are mostly involved with facilitation or induction of fluid intake (but inhibition may also be produced by α_1 adrenergic receptor activation) and forebrain α_2-adrenergic receptors are better characterized as involved with inhibition of both water and sodium intake [see Ferrari et al., 1991; Callera et al., 1993; Barbosa et al., 1995; De Luca Jr. et al, 1994; De Luca Jr. & Menani, 1997, for review]. The present chapter focuses on the role of α_2-adrenergic receptors, and the possible relationship of those receptors with imidazoline receptors, as assessed by pharmacological and functional studies, in the control of fluid intake.

The first part of this chapter is concerned with the characterization of the function of α_2-adrenergic receptors in the inhibition of fluid intake, the attempts to dissociate their function from the participation of imidazoline receptors and how the two receptors may interact. Then we focus on the effects of the anti-hypertensive mixed α_2-adrenergic/imidazoline receptor binding agonists moxonidine and clonidine on behavioral and renal responses related to fluid-electrolyte balance, leading to the novel finding that α_2-adrenergic receptors in the hindbrain have a facilitatory role in the control of fluid, particularly hypertonic NaCl, intake.

PARTICIPATION OF NORADRENALINE ACTING ON α_2-ADRENERGIC RECEPTORS IN THE INHIBITION OF FLUID INTAKE

Noradrenaline injected into the forebrain reduces (up to two hours) either thirst or sodium appetite specifically, apart from inducing a competing behavior, such as hunger, general depression or alterations in arterial pressure [Leite et al., 1992; De Luca Jr. et al., 1994; De Paula et al., 1996; Yada et al. 1997a; Sugawara et al., 1999]. Alpha$_2$-adrenergic/imidazoline receptor agonists injected into the forebrain produce similar specific effects and α_2-adrenergic receptor antagonists inhibit the effects of noradrenaline and of the other agonists on fluid intake generated by several types of stimuli [Fregly et al., 1981; Ferrari et al., 1990, 1991; Callera et al., 1993,1994; De Paula et al., 1996; Sato et al., 1996; De Luca Jr. & Menani, 1997; Yada et al. 1997a,b; De Luca Jr. et al. 1999; Menani et al., 1999; Sugawara et al., 1999; De Oliveira et al., 2003]. The effect of intracerebroventricular (icv) noradrenaline is also inhibited by icv L-type calcium channel blocker [De Luca Jr. et al., 2002], and likely dependent on activation of post-synaptic receptors. Pre-synaptic α_2-adrenergic receptors exert a negative feedback control on the synaptic release of noradrenaline [Langer, 1997]. However, those receptors are also located post-synaptically in the brain [Kalsner, 2001; French, 1995] and the inhibition that icv injection of clonidine induces on water and sodium intake is not reversed by prior icv injection of noradrenaline at low doses that do not alter these ingestive behaviors [Sugawara, 1999] (Figure 1). Therefore, the inhibition of fluid intake induced by noradrenaline is mostly dependent on post-synaptic action.

A physiological role of endogenous noradrenaline, and therefore of α_2-adrenergic receptors, in the inhibition of fluid intake has been hard to demonstrate. In several experiments performed in our laboratory, the central injection of only α_2-adrenergic receptor antagonists has hardly resulted in enhanced fluid intake, even at doses higher than the ones necessary to block the effects of agonists like clonidine or moxonidine [Yada et al. 1997b; Sugawara, 1999; de Oliveira et al., 2003]. In one experiment [Sugawara, 1999], the α_2-adrenergic/imidazoline receptor antagonist idazoxan (320 nmol/1 µl each injection) was injected icv 15 min prior and 75 min after allowing extracellular-dehydrated rats to have access to water and 0.3 M NaCl. Rats started to increase water intake 75 minutes after the access to fluids and there was a slight (33%) enhancement of water intake at 120 and 150 min of the test (Figure 2) and no effect on 0.3 M NaCl intake (not shown). Only an intermediate effective dose (40 nmol) of the α_2-adrenergic receptor antagonist RX 821002 injected icv produced an enhancement of similar magnitude in 0.3 M NaCl intake induced by 24 h of sodium depletion produced by subcutaneous (sc) injection of furosemide (20 mg/kg of body weight) plus 24 h of sodium deficient food [De Oliveira et al., 2003]. Single effective doses of the two α_2-adrenergic receptor antagonist yohimbine or idazoxan injected centrally had no effect on water deprivation-induced water intake or on sodium depletion-induced sodium appetite [Yada et al. 1997b]. Thus, it seems that central α_2-adrenergic receptors have a small, if any, participation in the satiating phase of fluid intake. Central injection of idazoxan also failed to reverse the anti-hedonic effect of quinine added to water in water deprived animals (Figure 3), suggesting that the inhibition induced by α_2-adrenergic receptor activation is not related to the production of an aversive taste [Sugawara, 1999].

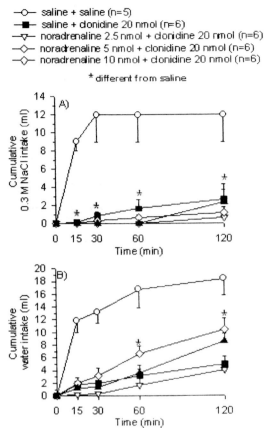

Figure 1. A) Cumulative 0.3 M NaCl intake of sodium depleted rats (diuretic furosemide – 20 mg/kg of body weight sc + 24 h of removal of ambient sodium), and B) cumulative water intake induced by 24 h of water deprivation. By the end of the 24 h, rats were treated with icv injections of saline or noradrenaline (2.5, 5 and 10 nmol/1 μl) + saline or clonidine (20 nmol/1 μl) prior to have access to fluids. The results are reported as mean ± SEM. Significant differences: p< 0.05. n = number of rats.

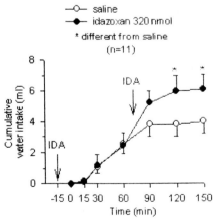

Figure 2. Cumulative water intake of rats that received one sc injection of the diuretic furosemide (20 mg/kg of body weight) 120 min before the access to water and 0.3 M NaCl (time 0). Food was removed before furosemide injection. Idazoxan (320 nmol/1 μl) or saline was injected icv at –15 and +75 min (arrows). The results are reported as mean ± SEM. Significant differences: p< 0.05. n = number of rats.

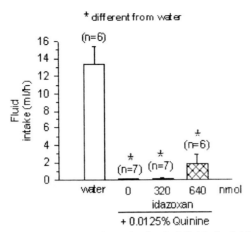

Figure 3. Water or 0.0125% quinine intake of rats deprived of fluids for 24 h. Animals received an icv injection of idazoxan (0, 320 or 640 nmol) 20 min prior to access to either fluid. The results are reported as mean ± SEM. Significant differences: $p < 0.05$. n = number of rats.

It is possible that the activation of central α_2-adrenergic receptors interact with the effects of other inhibitors of fluid intake. Idazoxan injected icv partially deactivates the inhibition of sodium appetite induced by central injection of oxytocin, and central clonidine at antidipsogenic doses enhances de content of atrial natriuretic peptide in the rat hypothalamus and olfactory bulb [Sato et al., 1997; Bastos et al., 2001].

ALPHA$_2$-ADRENERGIC AND IMIDAZOLINE RECEPTORS IN THE CONTROL OF FLUID INTAKE

Clonidine was the earliest α_2-adrenergic receptor agonist known to have an antidipsogenic effect and the deactivation of this effect by the alkaloid yohimbine injected systemically confirmed a participation of α_2-adrenergic receptors in the inhibition of thirst [Le Douarec et al., 1971; Fregly et al., 1983,1984a]. However, further works showed that this interpretation is not straightforward. When yohimbine was injected centrally it was not able to fully reverse the effect of clonidine [Ferrari et al., 1990]. Thus, part of the effect of systemic yohimbine could result from its hypotensive action, and the remaining antidipsogenic effect of clonidine when yohimbine was injected centrally could result from the participation of another type of receptor. An antagonist action of central yohimbine was also absent when clonidine was shown to inhibit sodium appetite [Yada et al., 1997 b].

The reports [Bousquet et al., 1992] that the lowering of blood pressure by central clonidine was a result of its action on receptors that differentially bind to imidazolines, but have no affinity to phenylethylamines, like catecholamines, prompted us to combine intraencephalic injections of several agonists with and without the imidazoline ring. Ligands at α_2-adrenergic receptors with no imidazoline characteristic were the unspecific noradrenaline and the selective α-methylnoradrenaline [Ernsberger et al., 1995]. Ligands with an imidazoline moiety and/or affinity, ranging from higher to lower, and with potential agonistic action on both receptors, were bromoxidine (UK14304), clonidine, moxonidine, guanabenz and agmatine, being the last two chemically related to guanidines [Ernsberger et al., 1995; Hieble & Ruffolo, 1995; Reis & Piletz, 1997; Dardonville & Rozas, 2004]. Histamine and the imidazole-4-acetic acid were used as ligands at imidazoline receptors with no affinity at α_2-adrenergic receptors [Ernsberger et al., 1995]. One can see at compiled data from our laboratory [De Paula et al., 1996; Yada et al., 1997a; Sugawara, 1999; Menani et al., 1999; Sugawara et al., 1999, 2001], that the compounds with imidazoline characteristics, but with affinities for α_2-adrenergic receptors, are the most effective (lower doses to produce maximum effects) to reduce either sodium appetite or thirst (Figure 4). Notice the near complete suppression of the behavior with only UK14304, clonidine or moxonidine and the absence of an effect of agmatine, imidazole-4-acetic acid and histamine. The results suggest that the imidazoline moiety increases the inhibitory action of α_2-adrenergic receptor ligands on fluid intake and that UK14304, clonidine and moxonidine share some characteristic in common the other ligands lack.

Compiled data of combined forebrain injections of the agonists and antagonists [Ferrari et al., 1990; Yada et al., 1997b; Sugawara, 1999; Menani et al., 1999; Sugawara et al., 1999, 2001; De Oliveira et al., 2003] also reinforce the importance of the imidazoline moiety for the inhibition of fluid intake (Figure 5). Yohimbine and the azepine SK&F86466 [Ernsberger et al., 1995; Hieble & Ruffolo, 1995] were weak antagonists even when the agonist was noradrenaline or the selective α_2-adrenergic receptor agonist α-methylnoradrenaline. The imidazolines idazoxan and its methoxy analogue RX 821002 [Ernsberger et al., 1995; Hieble & Ruffolo, 1995] were the most effective antagonists, and idazoxan was effective to inhibit even the effect of the non-imidazoline noradrenaline.

Although reinforcing the participation of imidazoline receptors, the results also point to α_2-adrenergic receptors as mediators of the inhibition of fluid intake. This is shown by the complete reversal of the effect of noradrenaline by idazoxan, by the partial effect of SK&F8646 on noradrenaline (sodium intake), and by the effects of yohimbine and SK&F86466 on moxonidine and clonidine. In addition, RX 821002 and UK14304 are considered respectively α_2-adrenergic receptor antagonist and agonist with low affinity at imidazoline receptors, at least in the brain, in spite of their imidazoline-like structures [Ernsberger et al., 1995; Hieble & Ruffolo, 1995; French, 1995; Eglen et al., 1998].

The difficulty to antagonize the effects of α-methylnoradrenaline with idazoxan and with SK&F86466 is puzzling. Alpha-methylnoradrenaline is considered a selective α_2-adrenergic receptor agonist [Ernsberger et al., 1995]. Perhaps the affinity of noradrenaline at both α_1 and α_2 sites may provide a clue. Prazosin, an α_1-adrenergic receptor antagonist, is able to partially antagonize the effects of clonidine on water or sodium intake [Ferrari et al., 1990; Yada et al., 1997b]. There are α_2-adrenergic receptor subtypes that bind to prazosin [French, 1995; Eglen et al., 1998]. Given that prazosin is not more effective than yohimbine or idazoxan to antagonize clonidine [Ferrari et al., 1990; Yada et al., 1997b] and given the effects of the other antagonists on clonidine shown here, then it is more likely that we are dealing with α_2-adrenergic receptor subtypes than with α_1-adrenergic receptors. Recall that the α_1 agonist phenylephrine, although much less potent than clonidine, also inhibits sodium and water intake [Ferrari et al., 1990; Callera et al., 1993; De Paula et al., 1996; Yada et al., 1997a]. Thus, noradrenaline would act on receptors that combine the two characteristics, but how much the effect of noradrenaline has to do with the effects of the imidazolines?

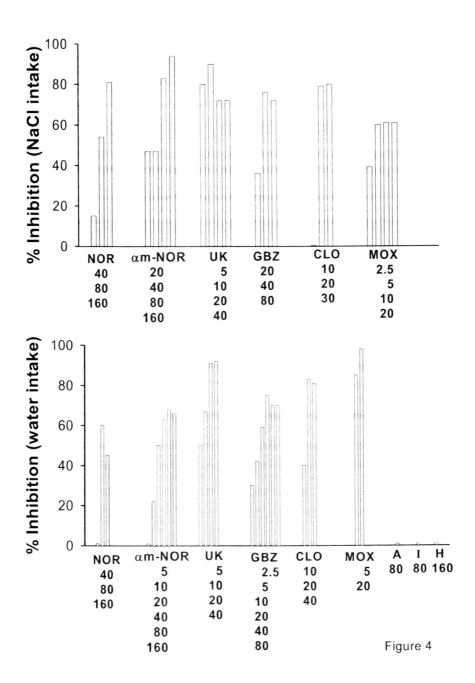

Figure 4. Compiled data showing the inhibition (% of control injected with vehicle) of NaCl and water intake by phenylethylamines, imidazolines and guanidines injected into the forebrain (see text for references). Noradrenaline (NOR), α-methylnoradrenaline (αm-NOR), UK14304 (UK), guanabenz (GBZ), clonidine (CLO), moxonidine (MOX), agmatine (A), imidazole-4-acetic acid (I) and histamine (H) were injected 15 to 20 min before starting the test of either NaCl or water intake. The numbers below each agonist correspond to the respective injected doses (nmol).

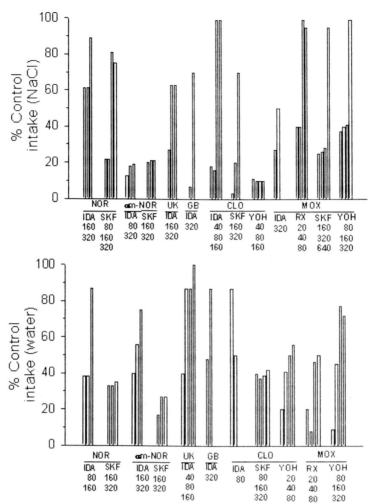

Figure 5. Compiled data showing the inhibition (% of control injected with vehicle) of NaCl and water intake by phenylethylamines, imidazolines and guanidines injected alone or combined with the antagonists into the forebrain (see text for references). The agonists noradrenaline (NOR, 80 nmol), α-methylnoradrenaline (αm-NOR, 80 nmol), UK14304 (UK, 10 nmol), guanabenz (GBZ, 40 nmol), clonidine (CLO, 20 nmol) and moxonidine (MOX, 20 nmol) were injected 15 to 20 min before starting the test of either NaCl or water intake. The antagonists idazoxan (IDA), SK&F 86466 (SKF), yohimbine (YOH) and RX 821002 (RX) were injected 15 to 20 min before the agonists. The numbers below each antagonist correspond to the respective injected doses (nmol).

The literature has emphasized that α_2-adrenergic and imidazoline receptors are distinct from each other [Ernsberger et al., 1995; French, 1995; Hieble & Ruffolo, 1995; Reis & Piletz, 1997; Bousquet et al., 1992, 2003], and therefore the effects of the agonists and antagonists, particularly of noradrenaline, on fluid intake are not necessarily on the same receptor. However, it seems that only the imidazoline property is not sufficient for an agonist effect on fluid intake considering the failure to produce any result with imidazole-4-acetic acid or histamine, differently from what these agonists do in other systems [Ernsberger et al., 1995; Prell et al., 2004]. A synergic interaction between α_2-adrenergic and imidazoline receptors has been proposed [Bousquet et al., 2003], which is perhaps a response to the controversial role of these receptors in the control of blood pressure [Ernsberger & Haxhiu, 1997; Guyenet, 1997]. Our data on fluid intake show that the most effective inhibitory response to α_2-adrenergic receptor activation depends on an imidazoline property and, thus, it also suggest that somehow the α_2-adrenergic and imidazoline receptors interact in either facilitatory or synergic way.

EFFECTS OF CLONIDINE AND MOXONIDINE ON FLUID INTAKE

Mixed α_2-adrenergic and imidazoline receptor agonists like clonidine and moxonidine are well known central acting anti-hypertensive drugs. Besides the anti-hypertensive action, clonidine and moxonidine injected in different forebrain sites, like the lateral ventricle (LV), third ventricle (3rd V), septal area, lateral preoptic area or lateral hypothalamus also strongly inhibit water intake induced by different stimuli [Le Douarec et al., 1971; Fregly et al., 1981, 1984a, b; Ferrari et al., 1990; Callera et al., 1993; De Paula et al., 1996; De Luca Jr. and Menani, 1997; Menani et al., 1999]. Moreover, moxonidine injected into the LV or 3rd V induces diuresis and natriuresis and inhibits sodium intake [Menani et al., 1999; Sugawara et al., 1999; De Oliveira et al., 2003, Penner and Smyth, 1994a, b, 1995]. Thus these mixed α_2-adrenergic and imidazoline receptor agonists may activate different mechanisms to reduce volume expansion and arterial pressure. This suggests that the therapeutic effects of these drugs may result from the combination of direct effects reducing sympathetic discharges on cardiovascular system and indirect effects reducing body fluid volume. However, a recent study from our laboratory has shown that activation of α_2-adrenergic receptors by injections of moxonidine into the lateral parabrachial nucleus (LPBN) enhances NaCl intake in rats, [Andrade et al, 2004], suggesting that α_2-adrenergic receptors may have opposite roles in the control of sodium and water intake according to their distribution in the brain of the rat.

In spite some controversies [Guyenet, 1997], the anti-hypertensive effects of α_2-adrenergic and imidazoline receptor agonists are suggested to be due to reduction of sympathetic activity that results from the activation of imidazoline receptors localized in the rostroventrolateral medulla [Bousquet et al., 1992, 2003; Ernsberger et al., 1993 a, b, 1997; Haxhiu et al., 1994]. The diuretic and natriuretic effects of moxonidine are also attributed to a central or peripheral action on imidazoline receptors and the central effects are dependent on the sympathetic system [Smyth and Penner, 1999]. However, the antidipsogenic and antinatriorexigenic effects of clonidine and moxonidine have been shown to depend mainly on the activation of central α_2-adrenergic receptors and their possible interaction with imidazoline receptors. Inhibition of either water or hypertonic NaCl intake dependent on α_2-adrenergic receptor activation has been demonstrated with injection of noradrenaline icv and injection of α_2-adrenergic/imidazoline agonists into the septal area, lateral preoptic area, and lateral hypothalamus [Ferrari et al., 1990; Callera et al., 1993; De Paula et al., 1996; De Luca Jr. and Menani, 1997; Sugawara et al., 1999; Menani et al., 1999; De Oliveira et al., 2003; Andrade et al., 2003].

Although moxonidine injected into LV induces diuresis and natriuresis and inhibits water and NaCl intake it produces no change in mean arterial pressure (MAP) and heart rate (HR), [Penner and Smyth, 1994a,b, 1995; Nurminem et al., 1998; Menani et al., 1999; Sugawara et al., 1999; Andrade et al., 2003; De Oliveira et al., 2003; Moreira et al., 2003]. On the contrary, when injected into the 4th V, the only well known effect of moxonidine is the reduction of MAP and HR, [Nurminem et al., 1998; Moreira et al., 2004]. In this chapter we present results showing that the renal and antidipsogenic effects of moxonidine are dependent on the forebrain, while the effects of moxonidine and clonidine on sodium intake are more complex with these drugs producing inhibition (forebrain or hindbrain) and facilitation (hindbrain).

The effects of moxonidine on renal excretion were tested with injections into the LV and 4th V and the effects of moxonidine or clonidine on water and sodium intake were investigated with injections subcutaneously (sc) or into the LV, 4th V, lateral parabrachial nucleus (LPBN) and lateral hypothalamus (LH). A possible interaction between serotonergic and adrenergic mechanisms of the LPBN in the control sodium intake is also demonstrated.

Effects of Subcutaneous Moxonidine on Water and Sodium Intake

The inhibition of water and NaCl intake by moxonidine and clonidine injected centrally at doses that range from 5 to 40 nmol are well known [Fregly et al., 1981, 1984a; Ferrari et al., 1990; Sato et al., 1996; De Paula et al., 1996; Yada et al., 1997a,b; De Luca and Menani, 1997; Menani et al., 1999; Sugawara et al., 1999; De Oliveira et al., 2003]. Peripheral injections of clonidine at the same doses injected centrally also reduces water intake induced by peripheral isoproterenol, hipertonic saline or ANG II administration [Fregly et al., 1981, 1984b]. In this chapter we present the effects of subcutaneous (sc) injections of moxonidine on central ANG II-induced water intake and sc moxonidine or clonidine on 24 h sodium depletion-induced sodium intake.

Male Holtzman rats weighing 300 to 320 g were housed in individual stainless steel cages with free access to normal sodium diet (Purina rat chow), tap water and 0.3 M NaCl. Rats were submitted to 24 h of sodium depletion produced by combining sc injection of the diuretic furosemide (20 mg/kg of body weight) and sodium deficient food (powdered corn meal, 0.001% sodium, 0.33% potassium) + water. In the next day rats received sc injections of vehicle (saline or acidified saline in the case of moxonidine), clonidine or moxonidine 15 min before having access to 0.3 M NaCl and water. The ingestion of 0.3 M NaCl and water was recorded at 15, 30, 60 and 120 min after the access to fluids. In a group of animals water intake was induced by icv injections of ANG II. These animals were anesthetized with ketamine (80 mg/kg of body weight) combined with xylazine (7 mg/kg of body weight) and placed in a Kopf stereotaxic instrument. Stainless steel 23 gauge cannulas were implanted into the lateral ventricle (LV, coordinates: 0.3 mm caudal to bregma, 1.5 mm lateral to the midline and 3.6 mm below the dura mater) and fixed to the skull using acrylic resin and small screws. Injections into LV were performed using a 10 µl Hamilton syringe connected by polyethylene tubing (PE10) to 30 gauge injection cannula (2 mm longer than the guide cannula implanted in the brain) and the volume injected into was 1 µl.

While clonidine injected sc reduced sodium depletion-induced sodium intake at the dose of 40 µg/kg b. w., [$F_{(2; 68)} = 47.95$, $P < 0.05$], (two-way ANOVA), moxonidine sc only reduced sodium depletion-induced sodium intake at the dose of 3,200 µg g/kg b.w. [$F_{(3, 36)} = 13.4$, $p < 0.05$] (Figures 6 and 7). In sodium depleted rats, clonidine (40 µg g/kg b. w.) sc also abolished water intake associated to sodium intake [$F_{(2; 68)} = 35.78$, $P < 0.05$], while moxonidine sc only reduced water intake associated to sodium intake at the doses of 800, 1,600 or 3,200 µg/kg b. w., [F(3, 36) = 8.7, p < 0.05], (Figures 6 and 7). Moxonidine at the dose of 3,200 µg/kg b. w., but not 1,600 µg/kg b. w. also reduced water intake induced by icv ANG II (50 ng/1 µl) [F(2; 68) = 12.7, P < 0.05], (Figure 8). Therefore, while moxonidine and clonidine injected into the lateral ventricle at the same low doses inhibit water and hypertonic NaCl intake in rats, the effective doses of this two drugs injected sc are strongly different. The differences between the doses of sc clonidine and moxonidine to inhibit water and NaCl intake are probably due to some difficulty that moxonidine has to access to the brain regions involved with the control of water and NaCl intake when injected peripherally.

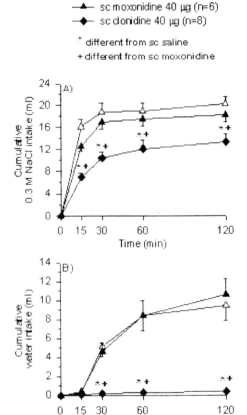

Figure 6. Cumulative 0.3 M NaCl (A) and its associated water (B) intake, induced by 24 h sodium depletion, in rats treated with sc injections of saline, moxonidine (40 µg/kg b. w.) or clonidine (40 µg/kg b. w.). The results are reported as mean ± SEM. Significant differences: p< 0.05. n = number of rats.

Comparative Effects of Clonidine and Moxonidine Injected into the Lateral and 4th Ventricles on Water and Sodium Intake and Renal Excretion

The α_2-adrenergic and imidazoline receptors are widely distributed in the central nervous system and may produce different responses depending on which brain areas they are acting [King et al., 1995; Macdonald and Scheinin, 1995; Ruggiero et al., 1998]. Reduction in sympathetic tone and decrease in arterial pressure and HR are produced by injections of moxonidine or clonidine into the 4th ventricle (4th V) and are suggested to depend on the activation of imidazoline receptors localized in the rostroventrolateral medulla (RVLM), [Haxhiu et al., 1994; Ernsberger et al., 1997]. On the other hand injections of α_2-adrenergic/imidazoline agonists into the LV inhibit water and NaCl intake and induce diuresis and natriuresis, but produce no cardiovascular effects. Although different studies have investigated the involvement of α_2-adrenergic/imidazoline receptors injected into LV in the control of water and 0.3 M NaCl intake and renal excretion, the possible effects of these drugs when injected into the 4th V were not investigated yet.

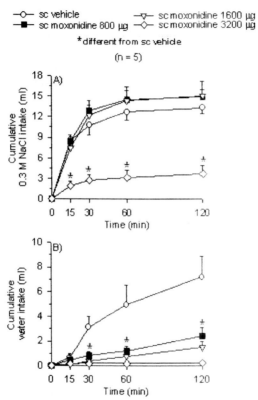

Figure 7. Cumulative 0.3 M NaCl (A) and its associated water (B) intake, induced by 24 h sodium depletion, in rats treated with sc injections of vehicle or moxonidine (800, 1600 and 3200 µg/kg b. w.). The results are reported as mean ± SEM. Significant differences: p< 0.05. n = number of rats.

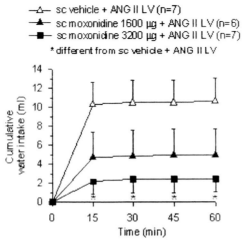

Figure 8. Cumulative water intake induced by icv (LV) injection of angiotensin II (ANG II, 50 ng/1 µl) in rats treated with sc injections of vehicle or moxonidine (1,600 and 3,200 µg/kg b. w.). The results are reported as mean ± SEM. Significant differences: $p < 0.05$. n = number of rats.

The effects of moxonidine and clonidine injected into the 4th V and the comparisons between the effects of these drugs injected into the 4th V and LV on water and 0.3 M NaCl intake and on renal excretion were investigated in male Holtzman rats. Rats weighing 300 to 320 g were housed in individual stainless steel cages with free access to normal sodium diet (Purina rat chow), tap water and 0.3 M NaCl. Stainless steel 23 gauge cannulas were implanted into the LV or into the 4th V (4th V coordinates: 13.3 mm caudal to bregma, in the midline and 6.4 mm below the dura mater) and fixed to the skull using acrylic resin and small screws. Injections were performed using a 10 µl Hamilton syringe and the volume injected was 1 µl.

In rats submitted to 24 h of sodium depletion, moxonidine (20 nmol/1 µl) injected into LV reduced 0.3 M NaCl intake for at least 2 h, while when injected into the 4th V it reduced the sodium depletion-induced 0.3 M NaCl intake only in the first hour of the test [$F_{(3, 128)}$ = 37.51; $P < 0.05$], (Figure 9A). No significant effect was observed on water intake in sodium depleted rats, [$F_{(3, 128)}$ = 1.81; $P > 0.05$], (Figure 9B). Moxonidine (20 nmol/1 µl) injected into LV also abolished 24 h of water deprivation-induced water intake [$F_{(3, 128)}$ = 43.7; $p < 0.05$], but did not modify water deprivation-induced water intake when injected into the 4th V (Figure 10).

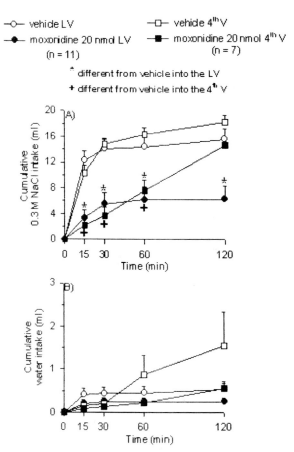

Figure 9. Cumulative 0.3 M NaCl (A) and its associated water (B) intake, induced by 24 h sodium depletion, in rats treated with injections of vehicle or moxonidine (20 nmol/1 µl) into LV or 4th V. The results are reported as mean ± SEM. Significant differences: $p < 0.05$. n = number of rats.

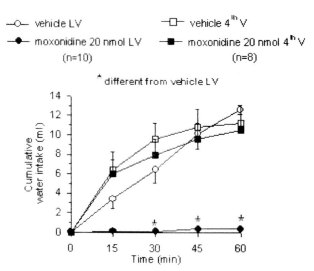

Figure 10. Cumulative water intake induced by 24 h water deprivation in rats treated with injections of vehicle or moxonidine (20 nmol/1 µl) into LV or 4th V. The results are reported as mean ± SEM. Significant differences: $p < 0.05$. n = number of rats.

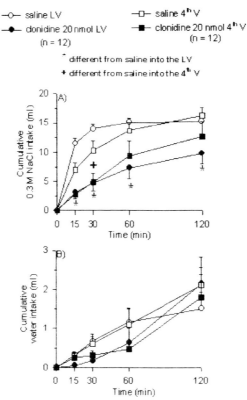

Figure 11. Cumulative 0.3 M NaCl (A) and its associated water (B) intake, induced by 24 h sodium depletion, in rats treated with injections of saline or clonidine (20 nmol/1 μl) into LV or 4th V. The results are reported as mean ± SEM. Significant differences: p< 0.05. n = number of rats.

Similar to moxonidine, clonidine (20 nmol/1 μl) injected into LV also reduced sodium depletion-induced 0.3 M NaCl intake throughout the sodium appetite test, while when injected into the 4th V it reduced 0.3 M NaCl intake only in the first 30 minutes of the test [$F_{(3, 176)}$ = 21.62; $P < 0.05$], (Figure 11A). Clonidine also produced no significant effect on water intake in sodium depleted rats, [$F_{(3, 176)}$ = 0.76; $P > 0.05$], (Figure 11B).

Renal excretion was tested in rats housed in metabolic cages that had food, not water removed 14 to 16 h before the test. After this period, rats were submitted to two gastric water loads (5% of body weight each one, with one-hour interval between them). Fifteen minutes before the second load, moxonidine (20 nmol/1 μl) or vehicle was injected into the LV or 4th V. Urine samples were collected every 30 min during 2 h starting immediately after the second load. Moxonidine (20 nmol/1μl) injected into the LV induced diuresis [$F_{(3, 144)}$ = 18.4; p<0.05] and natriuresis [$F_{(3, 144)}$ = 9.0; p<0.05], but did not alter K$^+$ excretion [$F_{(9, 144)}$ = 0.2; p>0.05], (Figure 12). Moxonidine injected into 4th V produced no alteration in urinary volume, Na$^+$ and K$^+$ excretion, (Figure 12).

Arterial pressure and HR were recorded in unanesthetized rats that had a polyethylene tubing (PE 10 connected to a PE 50) inserted into the abdominal aorta through the femoral artery and guided subcutaneously to the back of the rat on the day before the tests. Moxonidine (20 nmol/1 μl) injected into 4th V in normotensive rats (baseline MAP: 118 ± 2 mmHg and baseline HR: 375 ± 6 bpm) produced hypotension [$F_{(3, 60)}$ = 30.6; p<0.05],

(Figure 13A) and bradycardia [$F(3, 60) = 15.7$; $p<0.05$], (Figure 13B), whereas moxonidine injected into the LV did not affect MAP or HR.

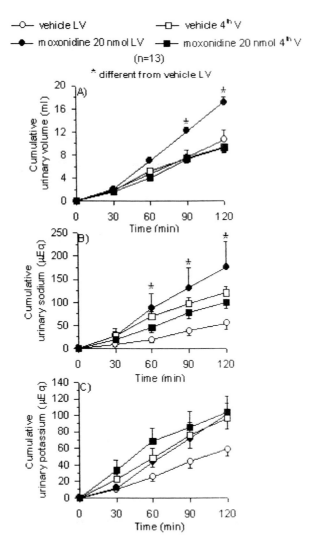

Figure 12. Cumulative urinary volume (A), sodium (B) and potassium (C) excretion in rats treated with injections of vehicle or moxonidine (20 nmol/1 µl) into LV or 4th V. The results are reported as mean ± SEM. Significant differences: $p< 0.05$. n = number of rats.

Therefore, moxonidine injected into the 4th V inhibited sodium depletion-induced sodium intake in the first hour of the sodium appetite test and clonidine inhibited sodium intake only in the first 30 min of test. Moxonidine into the 4th V had no effect on urinary Na^+, K^+ and volume excretion and on thirst produced by water deprivation. As previously demonstrated, moxonidine injected into the LV produced antinatriorexigenic, antipsogenic, diuretic and natriuretic responses. Moxonidine into the 4th V reduced MAP and HR, while into the LV produced no effect on MAP and HR as already known, [Nurminem et al., 1998; Moreira et al., 2004]. These results show that the effects of moxonidine into the 4th ventricle markedly contrast with those produced by LV injections.

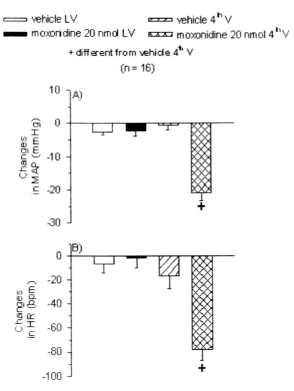

Figure 13. Changes on mean arterial pressure (A) and heart rate (B) in normotensive rats treated with injections of vehicle or moxonidine (20 nmol/1 μl) into LV or 4th V. The results are reported as mean ± SEM. Significant differences: p< 0.05. n = number of rats.

While the effects of moxonidine into the LV on sodium intake lasted for at least 2 h, moxonidine injected into the 4th V reduced sodium intake only in first hour of test, with animals recovering completely the intake at the end of 2 h. These results suggest that the hindbrain mechanisms are not so efficient to inhibit sodium intake. The inhibitory effect of moxonidine into the 4th V may be due to the activation of α_2-adrenergic/imidazoline receptors located in hindbrain areas like the area postrema (AP) and nucleus tractus solitarius (NTS). The α_2-adrenergic/imidazoline receptors have been shown to exist in the AP and NTS [King et al., 1995; Ruggiero et al., 1998] and drugs injected into the 4th V easily reach these areas. Moreover, lesions of the AP or of the AP and the adjacent NTS increase sodium intake [Contreras and Stetson, 1981; Kosten et al., 1983; Hyde and Miselis, 1984; Watson, 1985; Edwards et al.,1993], suggesting that inhibitory mechanisms to control sodium intake are present in these areas.

The inhibition of water intake and the natriuresis and diuresis to moxonidine was only produced by injections into the LV, which suggests that contrary to sodium intake these effects are exclusively due to the activation of forebrain α_2-adrenergic/ imidazoline receptors. Previous studies had already shown the antidipsogenic effects of LV moxonidine on water intake induced by 24 h water deprivation or central injection of ANG II and carbachol [Menani et al., 1999]. The renal effects of moxonidine into the LV were also previously demonstrated and they are likely due to reduced renal sympathetic discharge [Penner and Smyth, 1995]. The reduction in sympathetic activity is also the mechanism involved in the hypotension and bradycardia produced by moxonidine acting in the hindbrain or more specifically into the RVLM, [Ernsberger et al., 1994; Haxhiu et al., 1994; Ernsberger and Haxhiu, 1997; Khokhlova et al., 2001; Granata, 2004]. Therefore, a common mechanism, the reduction in sympathetic nerve discharge, is involved in the diuresis, natriuresis, hypotension and bradycardia produced by central moxonidine, but the central sites of control are completely different with the involvement of the forebrain in the diuresis and natriuresis and of the hindbrain in the cardiovascular responses.

Effects of Moxonidine and Clonidine Injected into the Lateral Hypothalamus on Water and Sodium Intake

Previous studies have shown that lesion of the lateral hypothalamus (LH) reduced or abolished sodium intake induced by sodium depletion or mineralocorticoid treatment [Wolf, 1967; Schulkin and Fluharty, 1985], suggesting that LH participates in the control of sodium intake. Clonidine injected into the LH reduced water deprivation and angiotensin II-induced water intake [Ferrari et al., 1990, 1991].

To compare the effects of clonidine and moxonidine injected into the LH on water intake and also tested the effects of these drugs into the LH on sodium depletion-induced 0.3 M NaCl intake. Male Holtzman rats weighing 280–320 g were submitted to the implant of a stainless steel cannula directed to the LH (LH, coordinates: 2.1 mm caudal to bregma, 1.3 mm lateral to the midline and 7 mm below the dura mater).

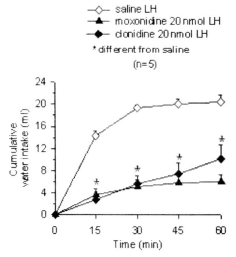

Figure 14. Cumulative water intake induced by 24 h water deprivation in rats treated with injections of saline, moxonidine (20 nmol/0.5 μl) or clonidine (20 nmol/0.5 μl) into LH. The results are reported as mean ± SEM. Significant differences: p< 0.05. n = number of rats.

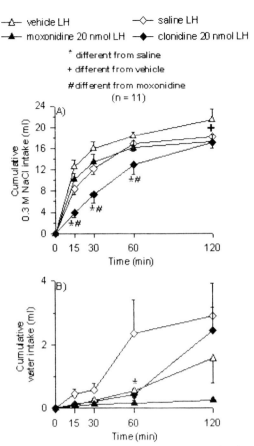

Figure 15. Cumulative 0.3 M NaCl (A) and its associated water (B) intake, induced by 24 h sodium depletion, in rats treated with injections of vehicle, saline, moxonidine (20 nmol/0.5 μl) or clonidine (20 nmol/0.5 μl) into LH. The results are reported as mean ± SEM. Significant differences: $p < 0.05$. n = number of rats.

Previous study already showed that injection of clonidine into the LH strongly reduced water deprivation-induced water intake [Ferrari et al., 1990]. Similar to clonidine, moxonidine (20 nmol/0.5 μl) injected into the LH reduced 24 h water deprivation-induced water intake [$F(2, 24) = 31,7$; $P < 0.05$], (Figure 14). Clonidine (20 nmol/0.5 μl) injected into the LH reduced sodium depletion-induced sodium intake during the first hour of test while moxonidine (20 nmol/0.5 μl) injected into the same area, only slightly reduced sodium intake in the last hour of test [$F(3, 40) = 6.12$, $P < 0.05$], (Figure 15A). Clonidine also reduced water intake associated to sodium intake at the time of 60 min [$F(3, 40) = 3.40$, $P < 0.05$], (Figure 15B). Therefore, similar to the studies of Ferrari et al., 1990, 1991, the present results show that the LH could be one of the sites for the action of α_2-adrenergic/imidazoline drugs to control water intake. In addition, clonidine into the LH also reduced sodium depletion-induced 0.3 M NaCl intake, while moxonidine into the LH at the dose used (20 nmol) did not affect 0.3 M NaCl intake.

Involvement of α_2-adrenergic Receptors in the Lateral Parabrachial Nucleus on Water and NaCl Intake

Inhibitory mechanisms for the control of water and NaCl intake have been demonstrated in the lateral parabrachial nucleus (LPBN). Bilateral LPBN injections of methysergide, a serotonergic receptor antagonist, markedly increase NaCl intake induced by ANG II administered either icv or into the subfornical organ (SFO), by 24 h of water deprivation, 24 h of sodium depletion, deoxycorticosterone acetate (DOCA), treatment with furosemide (FURO) + the angiotensin converting enzyme inhibitor captopril (CAP) injected subcutaneously [Colombari et al., 1996; Menani et al., 1996, 1998a; De Gobbi et al., 2000]. Besides serotonin, cholecystokinin (CCK) injected into the LPBN also inhibits NaCl and water intake [Menani and Johnson, 1998] in an interdependent and cooperative manner with serotonin in the LPBN [De Gobbi et al., 2001].

Recently we have shown that bilateral injections of moxonidine similar to the blockade of serotonin or cholecystokinin into the lateral parabrachial nucleus (LPBN) strongly increase 0.3 M NaCl and water intake induced by the treatment with FURO + CAP sc [Andrade et al., 2004]. The enhancement produced by moxonidine (up to ten fold the amount ingested by controls treated with FURO + CAP sc and vehicle into the LPBN) was completely suppressed by the α_2-adrenergic antagonist RX 821002.

In addition to the already published effects of moxonidine into the LPBN on FURO + CAP-induced water and NaCl intake [Andrade et al., 2004], in the present chapter we present the effects of bilateral injections of the selective α_2-adrenergic receptor agonist α-methylnoradrenaline and clonidine alone or combined with RX 821002 into the LPBN on the ingestion of 0.3 M NaCl and water induced by the treatment with FURO + CAP sc. These tests were performed in male Holtzman rats (290 to 310 g) that had bilateral stainless steel 23-gauge cannulas stereotaxically implanted in direction to the LPBN (coordinates: 9.4 mm caudal to bregma, 2.2 mm lateral to the midline and 4.3 mm below the dura mater). Water and 0.3 M NaCl were provided from burettes with 0.1-ml divisions that were fitted with metal drinking spouts. Water and 0.3 M NaCl intake were induced by the treatment with subcutaneous FURO (10 mg/kg of b. w.) + CAP (5 mg/kg of b. w.) as described previously [Fitts and Masson, 1989; Menani et al., 1996]. Rats received FURO + CAP treatment and were returned to their home cages in the absence of water and NaCl. Cumulative water and 0.3 M NaCl intakes were measured at 15, 30, 60, 90, and 120 min starting 1 h after FURO + CAP treatment when water and NaCl were available for animals. Bilateral injections of the agonists into the LPBN were performed 15 min before the access to water and 0.3 M NaCl. The antagonist (RX 821002) was injected 15 min before the agonist. At the end of the tests the brains were removed, fixed in 10% formalin, frozen, cut in 50-μm sections, stained with cresyl violet, and analyzed by light microscopy to confirm the injection sites into the LPBN.

Bilateral injections of clonidine (0.5, 1.0 and 5.0 nmol/0.2 μl) into the LPBN increased FURO + CAP-induced 0.3 M NaCl intake, [$F_{(3,12)}$ = 5.26; p<0.05], and water intake as showed by the significant interaction between treatments and time, [$F_{(12,84)}$ = 5.38; p<0.001], (Figure 16).

Bilateral injections of α-methylnoradrenaline (40 and 80 nmol/0.2 μl) also increased FURO + CAP-induced 0.3 M NaCl intake, [$F_{(2,16)}$ = 5.2; $P < 0.05$], (Figure 17A), while water intake increased only with the 40 nmol dose of α-methylnoradrenaline, [F(2,16) = 4.2; $P < 0.05$], (Figure 17B).

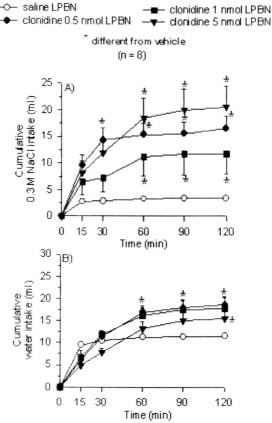

Figure 16. Cumulative 0.3 M NaCl (A) and water (B) intake, induced by sc FURO + CAP, in rats that received bilateral injections of clonidine (0.5, 1.0 or 5.0 nmol/0.2 µl) or vehicle into the LPBN. Results are expressed as means ± SE; n = number of rats.

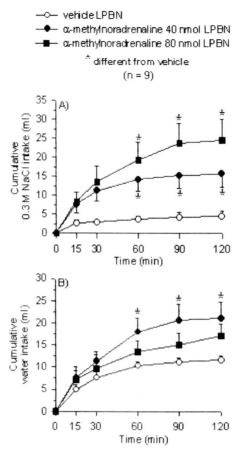

Figure 17. Cumulative 0.3 M NaCl (A) and water (B) intake, induced by sc FURO + CAP, in rats that received bilateral injections of α-methylnoradrenaline (40 or 80 nmol/0.2 μl) or vehicle into the LPBN. Results are expressed as means ± SEM; n = number of rats.

Previous injections of RX 821002 (160 nmol/0.2 μl) reduced the effect of α-methylnoradrenaline (80 nmol/0.2 μl) on 0.3 M NaCl intake, [$F_{(2,16)}$ = 6.7; $P < 0.05$], and on water intake, [$F_{(2,16)}$ = 9.4; $P < 0.05$], in the first 60 minutes test, (Figure 18).

The effects of clonidine and α-methylnoradrenaline injected bilaterally into the LPBN are similar to the effects of moxonidine into the LPBN. Bilateral injections of moxonidine into the LPBN enhanced in a dose-response manner FURO + CAP-induced 0.3 M NaCl intake. The enhancement produced by moxonidine (up to ten fold the amount ingested by controls treated with FURO + CAP sc and vehicle into the LPBN) was completely suppressed by RX 821002, an α2-adrenergic antagonist, [Andrade et al., 2004]. Although less intense, the effects of clonidine and α-methylnoradrenaline injected into the LPBN on water and NaCl intake, were similar to those produced by moxonidine.

The results presented in this chapter show that injections of clonidine and α-methylnoradrenaline into the LPBN similar to moxonidine into the LPBN (Andrade at al., 2004) increase FURO + CAP-induced sodium and water intake. In addition, the effect of α-methylnoradrenaline was also reversed by previous treatment with the α2-adrenergic receptor antagonist RX 821002. Considering that α-methylnoradrenaline binds specifically on α2-

adrenergic receptors and that its effect is reduced by previous injection of RX 821002, it is possible to conclude that the activation of LPBN α_2-adrenergic receptors facilitates NaCl and water intake.

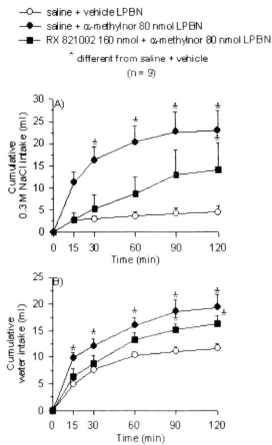

Figure 18. Cumulative 0.3 M NaCl (A) and water (B) intake, induced by sc FURO + CAP, in rats that received bilateral injections of RX 821002 (160 nmol/0.2 μl) or saline + α-methylnoradrenaline (80 nmol/0.2 μl) or vehicle into the LPBN. Results are expressed as means ± SEM; n = number of rats.

Although the activation of α_2-adrenergic receptors in the LPBN increases FURO + CAP-induced sodium and water intake, if rats were not treated with FURO + CAP, the activation of α_2-adrenergic receptors in the LPBN alone produces no effect on water and sodium intake [Andrade et al., 2004]. These results suggest that the activation of α_2-adrenergic receptors may block an inhibitory mechanism present in the LPBN allowing the increase in the ingestion of water and specially sodium induced by FURO + CAP. But only the blockade of the LPBN inhibitory mechanism by the activation of α_2-adrenergic receptors in the LPBN is not enough to stimulate sodium or water intake. The blockade of the serotonergic mechanism of the LPBN by bilateral injections of methysergide also increases stimulated sodium and water intake, but produces no effects on water and NaCl intake when the only treatment the animal receives is the bilateral injections of methysergide into the LPBN [Menani et al., 1996, 1998a,b]. Activation of α_2-adrenergic receptors in the LPBN also does not affect sucrose intake or arterial pressure which suggests that the effects of the activation of α_2-adrenergic receptors in the LPBN are not due to unspecific behavioral effects and also not related to any eventual activation of renin-angiotensin system as a consequence of hypotension [Andrade et al., 2004].

For many years, forebrain α_2-adrenergic/imidazoline receptors were suggested to have antidipsogenic effect [Le Douarec et al., 1971; Fregly et al., 1981, 1984a,b; Ferrari et al., 1990; Callera et al., 1993; De Paula et al., 1996; De Luca Jr. and Menani, 1997; Menani et al., 1999]. More recently, the inhibition of sodium intake by forebrain injections of α_2-adrenergic/imidazoline agonists was also reported [De Paula et al., 1996; Sato et al., 1996; Yada et al, 1997a,b; Sugawara et al., 1999; De Oliveira et al., 2003]. The results presented in this chapter show that clonidine and moxonidine injected into the 4th V also inhibit sodium intake, extending the existence of inhibitory mechanisms activated by α_2-adrenergic/imidazoline agonists also to the hindbrain. And, more interesting, the results also show that the activation of α_2-adrenergic receptors in the LPBN by injections of clonidine, moxonidine and α_2-methylnoradrenaline enhances an existing water and, specially, sodium intake. Therefore previous and the present results show that the activation of central α_2-adrenergic receptors can produce opposite effects on sodium and water intake depending on the site of action. The inhibitory effect of moxonidine injected into the 4th V on sodium intake was shorter (1 h) than the effects of injections into the LV (more than 2 h). One possibility to explain these differences is that moxonidine injected into the 4th V initially activate the inhibitory mechanisms for sodium intake and late it might reach the LPBN activating the facilitatory mechanisms, which would oppose the action of the inhibitory mechanisms.

Interaction between Serotonergic and α_2-adrenergic Mechanisms of the LPBN in the Control of Water and Sodium Intake

Previous studies have shown that the serotonergic $5HT_{2A/2C}$ agonist 2,5-dimetoxy-4-iodoamphetamine hydrobromide (DOI) injected bilaterally into the LPBN inhibits, while injections of methysergide (serotonergic receptor antagonist) into the LPBN increase sodium and water intake, suggesting the existence of important serotonergic inhibitory mechanisms in the LPBN controlling water and NaCl intake, [Menani et al., 1996]. The results presented in this chapter show that activation of α_2-adrenergic receptors in the LPBN increases sodium and water intake. To test a possible interaction between the serotonergic and α_2-adrenergic mechanisms in the LPBN in the control of water and NaCl intake, rats with stainless steel cannulas implanted bilaterally into the LPBN were treated with furosemide + captopril sc and bilateral injections of RX 821002 or moxonidine + DOI or methysergide into the LPBN.

Bilateral injections of the serotonergic agonist DOI (5 μg/0.2 μl) into the LPBN inhibited, while injections of moxonidine (5 nmol/0.2 μl) into the LPBN enhanced furosemide + captopril-induced 0.3 M NaCl intake, [$F_{(3,21)} = 12.3$; $p<0.01$], (Figure 19A). Combining DOI with moxonidine into the LPBN, the inhibitory effect of DOI was abolished and 0.3 M NaCl intake increased similar to moxonidine alone injected into the LPBN, (Figure 19A).

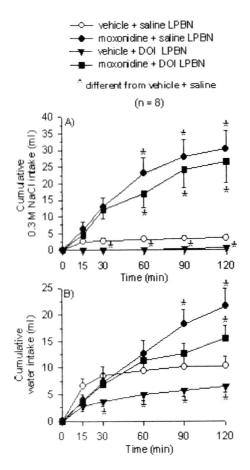

Figure 19. Cumulative 0.3 M NaCl (A) and water (B) intake, induced by sc FURO + CAP, in rats that received bilateral injections of moxonidine (0.5 nmol/0.2 μl) or vehicle + DOI (5 μg/0.2 μl) or saline into the LPBN. Results are expressed as means ± SEM; n = number of rats.

DOI into the LPBN also inhibited and moxonidine increased furosemide + captopril-induced water intake. Combining moxonidine and DOI into the LPBN, the effect of DOI on water intake was also abolished and water intake was similar to when moxonidine alone was injected into the LPBN, [F(3,21) = 6.08; p<0.05], (Figure 19B).

Bilateral injections of methysergide (4 μg/0.2 μl) into the LPBN increased 0.3 M NaCl intake [F(3, 21) = 4.14; p<0.05], and this effect of methysergide injected into the LPBN was not modified by previous injections of RX 821002 (20 nmol/0.2 μl) into the LPBN, (Figure 20A). In this group of rats, water intake was not significantly affected by any treatment, [F(3,21) = 0.15; p>0.05], (Figure 20B). The 20 nmol dose of RX 821002 is an effective dose to block the effects of moxonidine on water and NaCl intake [Andrade et al., 2004].

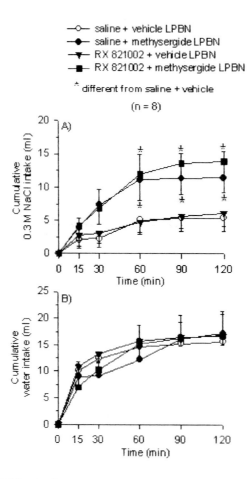

Figure 20. Cumulative 0.3 M NaCl (A) and water (B) intake, induced by sc FURO + CAP, in rats that received bilateral injections of RX 821002 (20 nmol/0.2 μl) or saline + methysergide (4 μg/0.2 μl) or vehicle into the LPBN. Results are expressed as means ± SEM; n = number of rats.

The results show that the activation of α_2-adrenergic receptors in the LPBN completely abolishes the inhibition of water and NaCl intake produced by the activation of the LPBN serotonergic mechanism. On the other hand the blockade of α_2-adrenergic receptors in the LPBN does not alter the effects of the blockade of the serotonergic mechanisms in the same area. Therefore, the activation of α_2-adrenergic receptors in the LPBN inhibits the effects of the activation of the serotonergic mechanisms of the LPBN, i.e., the inhibitory mechanism activated by serotonin in the LPBN is deactivated by α_2-adrenergic receptor activation in the same area. It is possible that the α_2-adrenergic and the serotonergic receptors are located in the same post synaptic neurons in the LPBN with each receptor producing opposite effects on the activity of these neurons. Another possibility is that the serotonergic and α_2-adrenergic receptors are localized in different neurons, but in this case the α_2-adrenergic receptors have to be present in neurons that are distal to the neurons that present the serotonergic receptors. The sole blockade of α_2-adrenergic receptors by injections of RX 821002 into the LPBN produces no change on furosemide + captopril-induced 0.3 M NaCl intake. This suggests that the activation of α_2-adrenergic mechanism in the LPBN is not necessary to induce fluid intake by this treatment but, given the strength of this mechanism, it is possibly recruited to attenuate the serotonergic mechanism and produce intense sodium appetite in a more critical situation.

CONCLUSION

A more clear general picture must still be ascribed to noradrenaline and a possible interaction between α_2-adrenergic and imidazoline receptors in the physiological control of water and salt intake, but the richness of effects of the adrenergic agonists suggest important roles for the neurotransmitter. Results from injections into the LV and 4th V suggest that the mechanisms activated by α_2-adrenergic/imidazoline receptor agonists to produce diuresis, natriuresis and antidipsogenic effects are present only in the forebrain. The effects of α_2-adrenergic/imidazoline receptor agonists on sodium intake are more complex and both inhibition and facilitation have been described with central injections of moxonidine and clonidine. The strength of the inhibition produced by the several agonists tested on both water and NaCl intake is related to the presence of the imidazoline moiety, but the agonists must bind to α_2-adrenergic receptors, otherwise no effect is observed. The inhibition of sodium intake may involve forebrain and hindbrain mechanisms, while facilitation depends on hindbrain, more specifically on the LPBN, the site where bilateral injections of moxonidine, clonidine and α-methylnoradrenaline strongly increase sodium intake probably due to the blockade of the LPBN serotonergic inhibitory mechanisms.

Certainly the central α_2-adrenergic receptors are chief mediators of most of the effects of noradrenaline and the α_2-adrenergic/imidazoline agonists described here. However, imidazoline receptors may play a facilitatory role in the α_2-adrenergic receptor activity, particularly in the inhibition of NaCl and water intake, by an yet unknown mechanism.

ACKNOWLEDGMENTS

We thank Silas Pereira Barbosa, Reginaldo da Conceição Queiróz and Silvia Fóglia for expert technical assistance, Silvana A. D. Malavolta for secretarial assistance, and Ana L. V. de Oliveira for animal care. We would like to thank also Solvay Pharma and Dr. P. Ernsberger for the donation of moxonidine and Dr. P. Hieble, from Smith Kline & Beecham, for the donation of SK&F86466. This research was supported by public funding from Fundação de Amparo à Pesquisa do Estado de São Paulo (FAPESP), Conselho Nacional de Pesquisa (CNPq), and PRONEX. The original research presented in this chapter was conducted by L. B. Oliveira, C. A. F. Andrade, and A. M. Sugawara, as partial fulfillment of the requirements for a master or doctoral degree at the Joint UFSCar/UNESP Graduate Program in Physiological Sciences. A. M. Sugawara is now at Universidade São Camilo and UNIFESP.

REFERENCES

Andrade, C. A. F.; Barbosa, S. P.; De Luca Jr, L. A. & Menani, J. V. (2004). Activation of α_2-adrenergic receptors into the lateral parabrachial nucleus enhances NaCl intake in rats. *Neuroscience, 129*, 25-34.

Andrade, C. A. F.; Oliveira, L. B.; Martinez, G.; Silva, D. C.; De Luca, L. A. Jr & Menani, J. V. (2003). Involvement of forebrain imidazoline and alpha(2)-adrenergic receptors in the antidipsogenic response to moxonidine. *Ann. N. Y. Acad. Sci., 1009*, 262-264.

Barbosa, S. P.; de Gobbi, J. I.; Zilioli L, Camargo, L. A.; Saad, W. A.; Renzi, A.; De Luca Jr, L. A. & Menani, J. V. (1995). Role of cholinergic and adrenergic pathways of the medial septal area in the water intake and pressor response to central angiotensin II and carbachol in rats. *Brain Res. Bull., 37*, 463-466.

Bastos, R.; Favaretto, A. L.; Gutkowska, J.; McCann, S. M. & Antunes-Rodrigues, J. (2001). Alpha-adrenergic agonists inhibit the dipsogenic effect of angiotensin II by their stimulation of atrial natriuretic peptide release. *Brain Res., 895*, 80-88.

Bousquet, P.; Feldman, J.; Tibiriça, E.; Bricca, G.; Greney, H.; Dontenwill, M.; Stutzmann, J. & Belcourt, A. (1992). Imidazoline receptors. A new concept in central regulation of the arterial blood pressure. *Am. J. Hypertens., 5*, 47S-50S.

Bousquet, P.; Greney, H.; Bruban, V.; Schann, S.; Ehrhardt, J. D.; Monassier, L. & Feldman, J. (2003). I(1) imidazoline receptors involved in cardiovascular regulation: where are we and where are we going? *Ann. N. Y. Acad. Sci., 1009*, 228-233.

Callera, J. C.; Camargo, L. A. A.; De Luca Jr., L. A.; Menani, J. V., Renzi, A. & Saad, W. A. (1993). Clonidine and phenylephrine injected into the lateral preoptic area reduce water intake in dehydrated rats. *Pharmacol. Biochem. Behav., 46*, 39-43.

Callera, J. C.; Saad, W. A.; Camargo, L. A.; Renzi, A.; De Luca Jr, L. A. & Menani, J. V. (1994). Role of the adrenergic pathways of the lateral hypothalamus on water intake and pressor response induced by the cholinergic activation of the medial septal area in rats. *Neurosci. Lett., 167*, 153-155.

Colombari, D. S. A., Menani, J. V. & Johnson, A. K. (1996). Forebrain angiotensin type 1 receptors and parabrachial serotonin in the control of NaCl and water intake. *Am. J. Physiol., 271*, R1470-R1476.

Contreras, R. J. & Stetson, P. W. (1981). Changes in salt intake after lesions of the area postrema and the nucleus of the solitary tract in rats. *Brain Res., 211*, 355-366.

Dardonville, C. & Rozas, I. (2004). Imidazoline binding sites and their ligands: an overview of the different chemical structures. *Med. Res. Rev., 24*, 639-661.

De Gobbi, J. I. F.; De Luca Jr, L. A. & Menani, J. V. (2000). Serotonergic mechanisms of the lateral parabrachial nucleus on DOCA-induced sodium intake. *Brain Res., 880*, 131-138.

De Gobbi, J. I. F.; De Luca, L. A. Jr; Johnson, A. K. & Menani, J. V. (2001). Interaction of serotonin and cholecystokinin in the lateral parabrachial nucleus to control sodium intake. *Am. J. Physiol., 280*, R1301-R1307.

De Luca Jr., L. A.; Camargo, L. A.; Menani, J. V.; Renzi, A. & Saad, W. A. (1994) On a possible dual role for central noradrenaline in the control of hydromineral fluid intake. *Braz. J. Med. Biol. Res., 27*, 905-914.

De Luca Jr, L. A. & Menani, J. V. (1997). Multifactorial control of water and saline intake: role of α_2-adrenoceptors. *Braz. J. Med. Biol. Res., 30*, 497-502.

De Luca Jr., L. A.; Nunes de Souza, R. L., Yada, M. M. & Meyer, E. W. (1999). Sedation and need-free salt intake in rats treated with clonidine. *Pharmacol. Biochem. Behav.*, 62, 585-589.

De Luca Jr., L. A.; Sugawara, A. M.; Pereira, D. T.; David, R. B. & Menani, J. V. (2002). Interaction between brain L-type calcium channels and alpha$_2$-adrenoceptors in the inhibition of sodium appetite. *Brain Res.*, 931, 1-4.

De Oliveira, L. B.; De Luca, L. A. & Menani, J. V. (2003). Moxonidine and central alpha$_2$ adrenergic receptors in sodium intake. *Brain Res.*, 993, 177-82.

De Paula, P. M.; Sato, M. A.; Menani, J. V. & De Luca Jr, L. A. (1996). Effects of central α-adrenergic agonists on hormone-induced 3% NaCl and water intake. *Neurosc. Lett.*, 214, 155-158.

Edwards, G. L.; Beltz, T. G.; Power, J. D. & Johnson, A. K. (1993). Rapid-onset "need-free" sodium appetite after lesions of the dorsomedial medulla. *Am. J. Physiol.*, 264, R1242-R1247.

Eglen, R. M.; Hudson, A. L.; Kendall, D. A.; Nutt, D. J.; Morgan, N. G.; Wilson, V.G. & Dillon, M. P. (1998). 'Seeing through a glass darkly': casting light on imidazoline 'I' sites. *Trends Pharmacol. Sci.*, 19, 381-390.

Ernsberger P. & Haxhiu, M. A. (1997). The I$_1$-imidazoline-binding site is a functional receptor mediating vasodepression via the ventral medulla. *Am. J. Physiol.*, 273, R1572-R1579.

Ernsberger, P.; Damon, T. H.; Graff, L. M.; Schäfer, S. G. & Christen, M. O. (1993a). Moxonidine, a centrally acting antihypertensive agent, is a selective ligand for I$_1$-imidazoline sites. *J. Pharmacol. Exper. Therap.*, 264, 172-264.

Ernsberger, P.; Elliot, H. L.; Weiman, H. J.; Raap, A.; Haxhiu, M. A.; Hofferber, E.; Low-Kroger, A.; Reid, J. L. & Mest, H. J. (1993b). Moxonidine: a second-generation central antihypertensive agent. *Cardiov. Drug Rev.*, 11, 411-431.

Ernsberger, P.; Friedman, J. E. & Koletsky, R. J. (1997). The I$_1$ – imidazoline receptor: from binding site to therapeutic target in cardiovascular disease. *J. Hypertension, 15 (suppl 1)*, S9-S23.

Ernsberger, P.; Graves, M. E.; Graff, L. M.; Zakieh, N.; Nguyen, P.; Collins, L. A.; Westbrooks, K. L. & Johnson, G. G. (1995). I1-imidazoline receptors. Definition, characterization, distribution, and transmembrane signaling. *Ann. N. Y. Acad Sci.*, 763, 22-42.

Ernsberger, P.; Haxhiu, M. A.; Graff, L. M.; Collins, L. A.; Dreshaj, I.; Grove, D. L.; Graves, M. E.; Schafer S. G. & Christen, M. O. (1994). A novel mechanism of action for hypertension control: moxonidine as a selective I$_1$-imidazoline agonist. Cardiovasc. *Drugs Ther.*, 8, 27-41.

Ferrari, A. C.; Camargo, L. A. A.; Saad, W. A.; Renzi, A.; De Luca Jr., L. A. & Menani, J. V. (1990). Clonidine and phenylephrine injected into the lateral hypothalamus inhibits water intake in rats. *Brain Res.*, 522, 125-130.

Ferrari, A. C.; Camargo, L. A. A.; Saad, W. A.; Renzi, A.; De Luca Jr., L. A. & Menani, J. V. (1991). Role of α_1- and α_2-adrenoceptors of the lateral hypothalamus in the dipsogenic response to central angiotensin II in rats. *Brain Res.*, 560, 291-296.

Fitts, D. A. & Masson, D. B. (1989). Forebrain sites of action for drinking and salt appetite to angiotensin or captopril. *Behav. Neurosci.*, 103, 865–872.

Fregly, M. J.; Kelleher, D. L. & Greenleaf, J. E. (1981). Antidipsogenic effect of clonidine on angiotensin II, hypertonic saline, pilocarpine and dehydration-induced water intake. *Brain Res. Bull., 7*, 661-664.

Fregly, M. J.; Rowland, N. E. & Greenleaf, J. E. (1983). Effects of yohimbine and tolazoline on isoproterenol and angiotensin II-induced water intake in rats. *Brain Res. Bull., 10*, 121-126.

Fregly, M. J.; Rowland, N. E. & Greenleaf, J. E. (1984a). A role for presynaptic α_2-adrenoceptors in angiotensin II-induced drinking in rats. *Brain Res. Bull., 12*, 393-398.

Fregly, M. J.; Rowland, N. E. & Greenleaf, J. E. (1984b). Clonidine antagonism of angiotensin-related drinking: a central site of action. *Brain Res., 298*, 321-327.

French, N. (1995). α_2-adrenoceptors and I_2 sites in the mammalian central nervous system. *Pharmac. Ther., 68*, 175-208.

Granata, A. R. (2004). Effect of moxonidine on putative sympathetic neurons in the rostral ventrolateral medulla of the rat. *Neurosignals, 13*, 241-247.

Grossman, S. P. (1962). Direct adrenergic and cholinergic stimulation of hypothalamic mechanisms. *Am. J. Physiol., 202*, 872-882.

Guyenet, P. G. (1997). Is the hypotensive effect of clonidine and related drugs due to imidazoline binding sites? *Am. J. Physiol., 273*, R1580-1584.

Haxhiu, M. A.; Dreshaj, I.; Schafer, S. G. & Ernsberger, P. (1994). Selective antihypertensive action of moxonidine is mediated mainly by I_1-imidazoline receptors in the rostral ventrolateral medulla. *J. Cardiovasc. Pharmacol., 24 (Suppl.1)*, S1-S8.

Hieble, J. P. & Ruffolo Jr., R. R. (1995). Possible structural and functional relationships between imidazoline receptors and alpha$_2$-adrenoceptors. *Ann. N. Y. Acad. Sci., 763*, 8-21.

Hyde, T. M. & Miselis, R. R. (1984). Area postrema and adjacent nucleus of the solitary tract in water and sodium balance. *Am. J. Physiol., 247*, R173-R182.

Kalsner, S. (2001). Autoreceptors do not regulate routinely neurotransmitter release: focus on adrenergic systems. *J. Neurochem., 78*, 676-684.

Khokhlova, O. N.; Murashev, A. N. & Medvedev, O. S. (2001). Role of I(1)-imidazoline receptors and alpha$_2$-adrenoceptors in hemodynamic effects of moxonidine administration into the rostroventrolateral medulla. *Bull. Exp. Biol. Med., 131*, 336-339.

King, P. R.; Gundlach, A. L. & Louis, W. J. (1995). Quantitative autoradiographic localization in rat brain of alpha$_2$-adrenergic and non-adrenergic I-receptor binding sites labeled by [^{3}H]rilmenidine. *Brain Res., 675*, 264-278.

Kosten, T.; Contreras, R. J.; Stetson, P. W. & Ernest, M. J. (1983). Enhanced saline intake and decrease heart rate after area postrema ablations in rat. *Physiol. & Beh., 31*, 777-785.

Langer, S. Z. (1997). 25 years since the discovery of presynaptic receptors: present knowledge and future perspectives. *Trends Pharmacol. Sci., 18*, 95-99.

Le Douarec, J-Cl.; Schmitt, H. & Lucet, B. (1971). Influence de la clonidine et des substances alpha-sympathomimétiques sur la prise d'eau chez le rat assoifé. *J. Pharmacol.(Paris), 2*, 435-444.

Leite, D. F.; Camargo, L. A.; Saad, W. A., Renzi, A.; Foglia, S.; De Luca Junior, L. A.; Menani, J. V. (1992). Role of cholinergic and adrenergic pathways of the medial septal area in the control of water intake and renal excretion in rats. *Pharmacol. Biochem. Behav., 42*, 1-8

MacDonald, E. & Scheinin, M. (1995). Distribution and pharmacology of alpha$_2$-adrenoceptors in the central nervous system. *J. Physiol. Pharmacol., 46*, 241-258.

Menani, J. V. & Johnson, A. K. (1998). Cholecystokinin actions in the parabrachial nucleus: effects on thirst and salt appetite. *Am. J. Physiol., 275*, R1431-R1437.

Menani, J. V., Sato, M. A., Haikel, L., Vieira, A. A., Andrade, C. A. F., Da Silva, D. C. F., Renzi, A. & De Luca Jr., L. A. (1999). Central moxonidine on water and NaCl intake. *Brain Res. Bull., 49*, 273-279.

Menani, J. V.; Colombari, D. S. A.; Beltz, T. G.; Thunhorst, R. L. & Johnson, A. K. (1998b). Salt appetite: Interaction of forebrain angiotensinergic and hindbrain serotonergic mechanisms. *Brain Res., 801*, 29-35.

Menani, J. V.; De Luca, L. A. Jr. & Johnson, A. K. (1998a). Lateral parabrachial nucleus serotonergic mechanisms and salt appetite induced by sodium depletion. *Am. J. Physiol., 274*, R555-R560.

Menani, J. V.; Thunhorst, R. L. & Johnson, A. K. (1996). Lateral parabrachial nucleus and serotonergic mechanisms in the control of salt appetite in rats. *Am. J. Physiol., 270*, R162-R168.

Moreira, T. S.; Takakura A. C.; Colombari, E.; De Luca Jr, L. A.; Renzi, A. & Menani, J. V. (2003). Central moxonidine on salivary gland blood flow and cardiovascular responses to pilocarpine. *Brain Res., 987*, 155-163.

Moreira, T. S.; Takakura, A. C.; Menani, J. V.; Sato, M. A.; Colombari, E. (2004). Central blockade of nitric oxide synthesis reduces moxonidine-induced hypotension. *Br. J. Pharmacol., 142*, 765-71.

Nurminen, M. L.; Culman, J.; Haass, M.; Chung, O. & Unger, T. (1998). Effect of moxonidine on blood pressure and sympathetic tone in conscious spontaneously hypertensive rats. *Eur. J. Pharmacol., 362*, 61-67.

Penner, S. B. & Smyth, D. D. (1994a). Sodium excretion following central administration of an I_1 imidazoline preferring agonist, moxonidine. *Br. J. Pharmacol., 112*, 1089-1094.

Penner, S. B. & Smyth, D. D. (1994b). Central and renal I_1 imidazoline preferring receptors: Two unique sites mediating natriuresis in the rat. *Cardiovasc. Drugs and Ther., 8*, 43-48.

Penner, S. B. & Smyth, D. D. (1995). The role of the peripheral sympathetic nervous system in the natriuresis following central administration of an I_1 imidazoline agonist, moxonidine. *Br. J. Pharmacol., 116*, 2631-2636.

Prell, G. D.; Martinelli, G. P.; Holstein, G. R.; Matulic-Adamic, J.; Watanabe, K. A.; Chan, S. L.; Morgan, N. G.; Haxhiu, M. A. & Ernsberger, P. (2004). Imidazoleacetic acid-ribotide: an endogenous ligand that stimulates imidazol(in)e receptors. *Proc. Natl. Acad. Sci. U S A., 101*, 13677-13682.

Reis, D. J. & Piletz, J. E. (1997). The imidazoline receptor in control of blood pressure by clonidine and allied drugs. *Am. J. Physiol. 273*, R1569-R1571.

Ruggiero, D. A.; Regunathan, S.; Wang, H.; Milner, T. A. & Reis, D. J. (1998). Immunocytochemical localization of an imidazoline receptor protein in the central nervous system. *Brain Res., 780*, 270-293.

Sato, M. A.; Sugawara, A. M.; Menani, J. V. & De Luca Jr., L. A. (1997). Idazoxan and the effect of intracerebroventricular oxytocin or vasopressin on sodium intake of sodium-depleted rats. *Regul. Pept., 69*, 137-142.

Sato, M. A.; Yada, M. M.; Renzi, A.; Camargo, L. A. A.; Saad, W. A.; Menani, J. V. & De Luca Jr, L. A. (1996). Antagonism of clonidine injected intracerebroventricularly in different models of salt intake. *Braz. J. Med. Biol. Res., 29*, 1663-1666.

Schulkin, J. & Fluharty, S. J. (1985). Further studies on salt appetite following lateral hypothalamic lesions: Effects of preoperative alimentary experiences. *Behav. Neurosci., 99*, 929-935.

Smyth, D. D. & Penner, S. B. (1999). Peripheral and central imidazoline receptor-mediated natriuresis in the rat. *Ann. N. Y. Acad. Sci., 881*, 344-357.

Sugawara, A. M. (1999). Adrenergic participation in hydro-saline intake: mechanisms and physiological role (Portuguese). Master Dissertation presented at the Graduate Program in Physiological Sciences at the Federal University of São Carlos (UFSCar).

Sugawara, A. M.; Miguel, T. T.; De Oliveira, L. B.; Menani, J. V. & De Luca Jr., L. A. (1999). Noradrenaline and mixed α_2 adrenoreceptor/imidazoline-receptor ligands: effects on sodium intake. *Brain Res., 839*, 227-234.

Sugawara, A. M.; Miguel, T. T.; Pereira, D. T. B.; Menani, J. V. & De Luca Jr., L. A. (2001). Effects of central imidazolinergic and alpha$_2$-adrenergic activation on water intake. *Braz. J. Med. Biol. Res., 34*, 1185-1190.

Watson, W. E. (1985). The effect of removing area postrema on the sodium and potassium balances and consumptions in the rat. *Brain Res., 359*, 224-232.

Wolf, G. (1967). Hypothalamic regulation of sodium intake: Relations to preoptic and tegmental function. *Am. J. Physiol., 213*, 1433-1438.

Yada, M. M.; De Paula, P. M.; Menani, J. V. & De Luca Jr, L. A. (1997a). Central α-adrenergic agonists and need-induced 3% NaCl and water intake. *Pharmacol. Biochem. Behav., 57*, 137-143.

Yada, M. M.; De Paula, P. M.; Menani, J. V.; Renzi, A.; Camargo, L. A. A.; Saad, W. A. & De Luca Jr, L. A. (1997b). Receptor-mediated effects of clonidine on need-induced 3% NaCl and water intake. *Brain Res. Bull., 42*, 205-209.

In: New Trends in Brain Research
Editor: F. J. Chen, pp. 127-142

ISBN 1-59454-834-X
© 2006 Nova Science Publishers, Inc.

Chapter VI

STIMULANT AND DEPRESSANT BEHAVIORAL ACTIONS OF ALCOHOL IN NON-SELECTED WISTAR RATS

*Fabiola Hernández-Vázquez and Milagros Méndez**

Departamento de Neuroquímica, Subdirección de Investigaciones Clínicas, Instituto
Nacional de Psiquiatría Ramón de la Fuente, Calzada México Xochimilco,
México D.F., Mexico

ABSTRACT

Low doses of alcohol have been reported to induce psychomotor activation in rodents, whereas high doses produce sedation. However, locomotor responses to alcohol may be influenced by different factors, including the dose and route of administration, the duration of drug exposure, the distinct sensitivity of rodent strains, the light-dark cycle and stressful situations. The aim of this work was to investigate locomotor responses in Wistar rats in normal and reverse light-dark cycles, as well as the effect of different doses of alcohol. Behavioral responses were assessed in an activity meter and scores of slow and fast horizontal movements, as well as slow and fast stereotyped movements were recorded. Rats were habituated for 30 min, then received an intraperitoneal (i.p.) saline injection and saline or alcohol was administered (0.25, 1 or 2.5 g/kg i.p.) after 30 min. A control group of animals was registered but not injected. Animals in the reverse light-dark cycle exhibited a higher motor response than those in the normal cycle. Thus, behavioral responses to alcohol were studied in reverse cycle animals. Forty four and 49 % significant decreases in total horizontal movements were observed in response to alcohol at doses of 0.25 and 2.5 g/kg, respectively, versus the control group. In contrast, a 69 % increase was found with 1 g/kg versus the saline group. This dose also increased total stereotyped movements by 41 and 92 % versus the control and saline groups,

* Corresponding author : Dr. Milagros Méndez. Tel. : (52) 56 55 28 11, ext. 212; Fax : (52) 55 13 37 22; Email
adress : ubach@imp.edu.mx

respectively, whereas a dose of 2.5 g/kg induced a 38 % decrease versus the control group. Total activity (total horizontal movements plus total stereotyped movements) was significantly increased (40 %) and decreased (43 %) by alcohol doses of 1 and 2.5 g/kg, respectively, versus the control group. The stimulant effect of alcohol was even higher (a 78 % increase) when compared to the saline group. Opposite behavioral alcohol effects were observed, 1 g/kg stimulating motor activity and 2.5 g/kg exhibiting a sedative effect. Our results suggest that stimulant alcohol effects may be mainly due to fast horizontal and fast stereotyped movements. In contrast, the sedative alcohol effects may involve similar contributions of slow and fast horizontal, as well as fast stereotyped movements. Alcohol behavioral effects may be closely related to activation of brain dopaminergic circuits.

INTRODUCTION

Alcohol consumption affects several biological functions and induces important behavioral changes, which are associated with alterations in several neuronal systems. Activation of brain dopaminergic pathways is involved in actions elicited by drugs of abuse, including alcohol. The dopaminergic mesocorticolimbic system plays an important role in the development of the positive reinforcing and rewarding actions of alcohol, which may lead to addictive behavior [34, 63]. Otherwise, alcohol also affects dopaminergic neurotransmission in the nigrostriatal pathway [21, 55], which may be implicated in determining brain sensitivity to alcohol [66]. Alcohol also interacts with other neurotransmitter and neuromodulator systems, including glutamate [29], serotonin [7], γ-aminobutyric acid (GABA) [57] and opioid peptides [26]. These interactions may contribute to the positive reinforcing actions of the drug.

Alcohol affects several neurobiological processes, such as temperature regulation, sleep and motor coordination [46]. Alcohol decreases body temperature and severe intoxication in a cold environment has been suggested to produce life-threatening declines in temperature (hypothermia). In addition, alcohol interferes with normal sleep patterns. Low doses of alcohol produce sleepiness and suppression of rapid eye-movement (REM) sleep. Chronic alcohol consumption may result in the loss of muscular coordination, which may be associated with peripheral neuropathy, a disorder commonly seen in alcoholics [46]. These data indicate that alcohol consumption may have serious repercussions in the functioning of the entire nervous system.

Alcohol exhibits biphasic behavioral effects in animals and humans. Low doses of alcohol have been reported to induce locomotor stimulation in most mouse [6] and some rat [28] strains, as well as psychomotor activation and euphoria in humans [41]. In contrast, high doses of alcohol decrease locomotor activity in mice and rats, and induce sedation in both animals and humans [17, 18]. Important conclusions on the biphasic effects of alcohol on locomotor activity have been provided by studies using animal models. However, conflicting data have been reported. Waller et al. (1986) [62] have shown that alcohol doses of 0.12 to 0.25 g/kg increase locomotor activity in alcohol preferring (P) inbred line of rats, while alcohol non-preferring (NP) animals failed to show increases in locomotor activity at any alcohol dose tested. Other studies have reported that alcohol doses of 0.12 to 0.5 g/kg do not affect locomotor activity in P, NP or Fawn-Hooded (FH) rats, whereas a dose of 1g/kg diminish motor activity in FH rats, as well as in Flinders Sensitive Line (FSL) and Flinders Resistant Line (FRL) rats [11]. In addition, Imperato and Di Chiara (1986) [31] reported increases and decreases in locomotor activity with doses of alcohol of 0.5 and 1 g/kg, respectively, in Sprague Dawley rats. Similar results were obtained by Schaeffer et al. (1988) [58], who reported a reduction in motor activity with a dose of alcohol of 1g/kg in the same strain of rats. Koros et al. (1998, 1999) [37, 38] did not observe a positive correlation between alcohol intake and locomotor activity in Wistar rats. These data indicate that alcohol's actions on locomotor activity may be importantly influenced by several factors, including the alcohol dose and the rodent strain used. The route of administration and the duration of alcohol exposure [47] may also contribute to the behavioral responses elicited by the drug.

Stress situations and light-dark cycle conditions may also affect the behavioral responses to alcohol. Studies in animals have suggested a close relationship between alcohol and stress. For instance, alcohol-seeking behavior is restored in abstinent rats by a stressor (an electrical shock in their feet) [40]. In humans, a positive correlation between stress and alcohol consumption has been observed, since alcohol intake relieves anxiety and helps people with stressful situations [50]. Other studies have shown that some stressors (i.e., a novel environment or a tail pinch) and alcohol administration increase locomotor activity in animals [2, 19, 52]. On the other hand, alcohol sensitivity is altered according to the light-dark phase during which the drug is consumed [24, 25]. Reinberg (1992) [51] has shown that the same dose of alcohol in human drinkers produces different effects depending on the hour of the day alcohol is ingested. In animals, this behavior is also observed. Animals consume more alcohol in the dark compared with the light phase of the day [25] and the absorption and elimination of alcohol is faster when the drug is consumed at midnight [24]. In addition, stress and circadian rhythms are closely linked, since higher responses to stressors (food restriction) are observed in the morning [56]. Thus, stressful and light-dark cycle conditions are critical in determining alcohol sensitivity and responsiveness, which may reflect differential behavioral responses. These factors may specifically affect different features of locomotor activity. Therefore, the aim of this work was to study the patterns of locomotor activity in non-selected Wistar rats in normal and reverse light-dark cycles. We investigated the effects of different doses of alcohol on motor activity as well, since alcohol dose-response studies have provided conflicting data.

MATERIALS AND METHODS

Animals

Male Wistar rats (200 - 300g) were housed five per cage and maintained in a 12h normal cycle (lights on at 7:00 h) (group A) or reverse cycle (lights on at 19:00 h) (group B). Rats of group B were changed to the reverse cycle one week before activity recording and were tested with red light. All animals had free access to standard laboratory chow and water (except during the test) and were habituated to the test room for 1 h. Experiments were conducted between 10:00 and 14:00 h.

Locomotor Activity Test

Locomotor activity was measured in an activity meter (Panlab, s.I., Letica Scientific Instruments) provided with a 45 x 45 cm arena and 16 infra-red beams, which are intended to measure forward locomotion by beam interruption. Locomotor activity was defined as the distance (number of beam interruptions) traveled by the rat during the 30 min test session at 2 min intervals. The activity meter was set to measure fast (F-MOV) and slow (S-MOV) horizontal movements and fast (F-STE) and slow (S-STE) stereotyped movements.

Normal and Reverse Cycle Experiments

Motor activity was measured in rats in normal or reverse light-dark cycles in 30 min sessions and records were compared.

Alcohol Administration and Activity Experiments

Animals in the reverse light-dark cycle were tested with different doses of alcohol, since their motor activity was higher than in the normal cycle rats. Animals were placed in the activity meter for a period of 30 min in order to habituate them to the testing environment (habituation phase). Then, all animals received an intraperitoneal (i.p.) saline injection with the purpose of diminish stress and activity was measured during 30 min (saline phase). Finally, animals received an i.p. injection of saline or alcohol (0.25, 1 or 2.5 g ethanol per kg) and activity was monitored for a period of 1 h (drug phase). Two control groups were included in the study, one receiving saline solution during the drug phase (saline group), the other not injected but recorded during the whole experiment (2 h) (control group).

Statistical Analyses

Statistical differences between animal groups in the normal and reverse cycles were determined by one way ANOVA. In alcohol administration experiments data were also analyzed by ANOVA, considering differences between alcohol doses tested and control groups. Significant differences between groups were investigated by the post hoc Tuckey-HSD test.

RESULTS

Motor Activity in Normal and Reverse Cycle Rats

Highest activity scores in all animals were observed during the first 10 min. Exploratory behavior and stereotyped movements were higher in animals in reverse than those in normal cycle. These differences were higher in fast horizontal (F-MOV) (Figure 1A) and fast stereotyped movements (F-STE) (Figure 1C) than in slow horizontal (S-MOV) and slow stereotyped movements (S-STE) (Figures 1B and 1D). Significant differences in F-MOV between normal and reverse cycle animals were only observed during the first 10 min (Figure 1A), whereas differences in S-SMOV, S-STE and F-STE were observed almost in the whole 30 min recording activity period (Figures 1B, 1C and 1D). Cumulated activity scores (beam interruptions) in 10 or 30 min periods in reverse compared with normal cycle animals showed significant increases of 51 and 72 % in F-MOV, 22 and 39 % in S-MOV, 46 and 53 % in F-STE and 8 and 24 % in S-STE (Figures 1A, 1B, 1C and 1D, inserts).

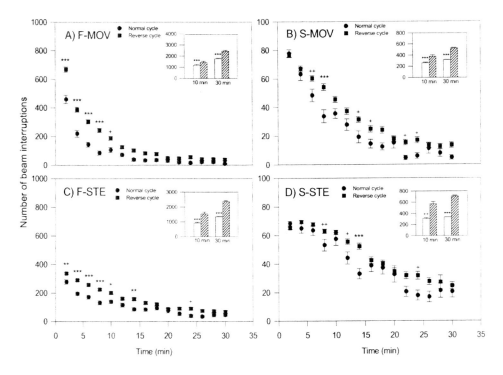

Figure 1. Time course of motor activity in normal and reverse cycle rats. F-MOV (A), S-MOV (B), F-STE (C) and S-STE (D) were measured in 2 min intervals during 30 min. Data represent the mean ± S.E.M. of 25 (normal cycle) or 30 (reverse cycle) animals. Activity is also shown as cumulated scores in the first 10 min of the test and total activity in 30 min (inserts). Inserts : white bars = normal cycle; hatched bars = reverse cycle. ***p < 0.0001; **p < 0.001; *p < 0.005; ++ p < 0.01; + p < 0.05.

Total horizontal activity (fast plus slow horizontal movements), total stereotyped movements (fast plus slow stereotyped movements) and total activity (total horizontal activity plus total stereotyped movements) were higher in rats in reverse cycle than in animals in normal cycle (Figures 2A, 2B and 2C). Cumulated scores in 10 or 30 min periods in reverse compared with normal cycle animals showed significant increases of 40 and 65 % in total horizontal activity, 36 and 45 % in total stereotyped movements and 41 and 52 % in total activity (Figures 2A, 2B and 2C, inserts).

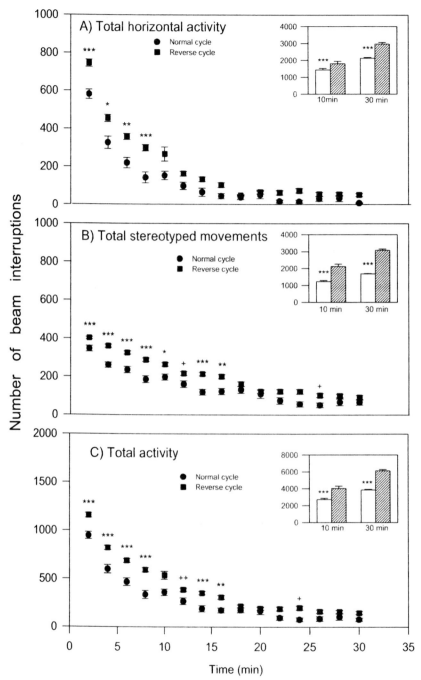

Figure 2. Time course of total motor activity in normal and reverse cycle rats. Total horizontal activity (A), total stereotyped movements (B) and total activity (C) were measured in 2 min intervals during 30 min. Data represent the mean ± S.E.M. of 25 (normal cycle) or 30 (reverse cycle) animals. Activity is also shown as cumulated scores in the first 10 min of the test and total activity in 30 min (inserts). Inserts : white bars = normal cycle; hatched bars = reverse cycle. ***$p < 0.0001$; **$p < 0.001$; *$p < 0.005$; ++$p < 0.01$; +$p < 0.05$.

Effect of Different Doses of Alcohol on Motor Activity

Habituation Phase

Since reverse cycle animals exhibited higher motor activity than those in normal cycle, we investigated the effect of different doses of alcohol in reverse cycle rats. No significant differences were observed in all activity parameters studied (F-MOV, S-MOV, F-STE and S-STE) during the habituation period (data not shown).

Saline Phase

Saline injection after a 30 min habituation period did not produce differences in F-MOV between animal groups (Figure 3). Saline injection decreased F-MOV when compared with the control (non-injected) group, although this difference was not significant (Figure 3). No significant differences were observed when examining S-MOV, F-STE and S-STE (data not shown).

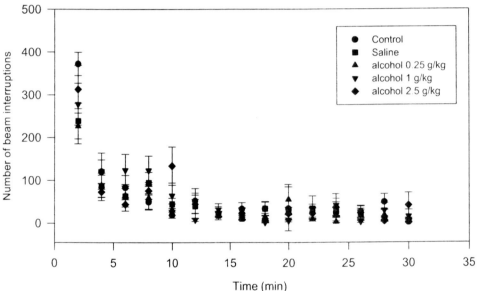

Figure 3. Effect of a saline injection on horizontal fast movements in reverse cycle rats. Animals were divided in 4 groups, which were subsequently re-injected with saline or alcohol at doses of 0.25, 1 or 2.5 g/kg. An additional non-injected group (control) was examined. Data represent the mean ± S.E.M. of 9 (control), 10 (saline), 9 (0.25 g/kg), 10 (1 g/kg) and 11 (2.5 g/kg) animals.

Drug Phase

Since the effects of different doses of alcohol were only significant during the first four intervals (8 min), results are presented as cumulated scores in 8 min. An alcohol dose of 1g/kg significantly increased F-MOV by 90 % when compared with saline-injected animals, but not with the control group. In contrast, alcohol doses of 0.25 and 2.5 g/kg were not significantly different from the saline group, but decreased F-MOV by 58 and 63 % respectively, when compared with the control group (Figure 4A). Significant differences were detected between alcohol groups : 186 and 226 % increases in F-MOV were observed when comparing 0.25 versus 1 g/kg and 2.5 g/kg versus 1 g/kg, respectively (Figure 4A). Alcohol at doses of 0.25, 1 or 2.5 g/kg did not significantly affect S-MOV, F-STE or S-STE, although the dose of 2.5 g/kg decreased S-MOV and F-STE by 46 %. An alcohol dose of 1 g/kg increased S-SMOV by 107 % compared with the dose of 2.5 g/kg (Figures 4B, 4C and 4D). Fast stereotyped movements were 86 % higher in response to an alcohol dose of 1 g/kg than the dose of 2.5 g/kg (Figure 4C). Since no significant differences were observed between the different groups of animals during the saline phase of the experiment (Figure 3), the observed effects during the drug phase are due to alcohol administration and not to a stress response (i.p. saline injection).

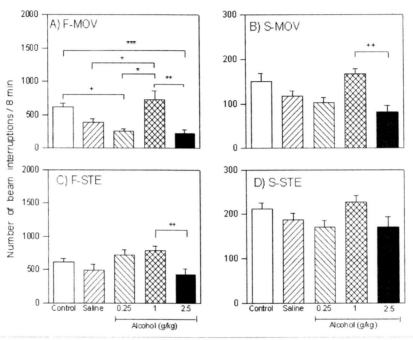

Figure 4. Effect of different doses of alcohol on horizontal activity and stereotyped movements in reverse cycle rats. Cumulated scores in 8 min are shown for F-MOV (A), S-MOV (B), F-STE (C) and S-STE (D). Data represent the mean ± S.E.M. of 9 (control), 10 (saline), 9 (0.25 g/kg), 10 (1 g/kg) and 11 (2.5 g/kg) animals. *** $p < 0.001$; ** $p < 0.005$; * $p < 0.01$; [+] $p < 0.05$.

Alcohol administered at doses of 0.25 and 2.5 g/kg significantly decreased total horizontal activity by 44 and 49 % in comparison with the control group (Figure 5A). In contrast, a dose of 1g/kg significantly increased total horizontal activity when compared with all groups tested : 69 % (saline), 117 % (0.25 g/kg) and 141 % (2.5 g/kg), except with the control group (Figure 5A). Alcohol at the same dose (1 g/kg) significantly increased total stereotyped movements when compared with all groups tested : 41 % (control), 92 % (saline), 51 % (0.25 g/kg) and 129 % (2.5 g/kg). A dose of 2.5 g/kg significantly decreased total stereotyped movements by 38 % versus the control group (Fig 5B). Alcohol at a dose of 1g/kg also increased total activity when compared with all groups tested : 40 % (control), 78 % (saline), 97 % (0.25 g/kg) and 150 % (2.5 g/kg), whereas a dose of 2.5g/kg decreased total activity by 43% when compared with the control group. Total activity was not significantly affected by an alcohol dose of 0.25g/kg (Figure 5C). No significant differences were observed between the saline and control groups (Figures 4 and 5).

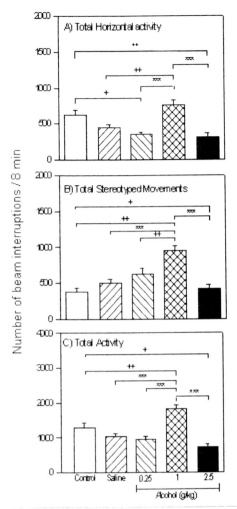

Figure 5. Effect of different doses of alcohol on total motor activity in reverse cycle rats. Cumulated scores in 8 min are shown for total horizontal activity (A), total stereotyped movements (B) and total activity (C). Data represent the mean ± S.E.M. of 9 (control), 10 (saline), 9 (0.25 g/kg), 10 (1 g/kg) and 11 (2.5 g/kg) animals. *** $p < 0.0001$; ** $p < 0.01$, * $p < 0.05$.

DISCUSSION

Alcohol doses with stimulant properties are difficult to establish in humans, since the same dose may have stimulant or depressant effects in different subjects [15, 16]. This difference is also seen in animals, given that there are several factors that affect the behavioral responses to alcohol. In this study, we have shown that alcohol, at a dose of 1g/kg, increased total horizontal activity and total stereotyped movements in non-selected Wistar rats. A slight but not significant increase in locomotor activity in Wistar rats has also been reported in response to the same dose of alcohol [45]. In contrast, this alcohol dose has been reported to decrease locomotor activity and to induce sedation in Sprague-Dawley rats [31, 58], as well as in FH, FSL and FRL strains of rats, with no effect in P and NP rats [11]. A depressant effect of an alcohol dose of 1 g/kg was also reported by Gingras and Cools (1996) [28] in selected Nijmegen Wistar rats. Stimulant alcohol effects have been obtained with lower doses (0.1 - 0.5 g/kg i.p.) [11, 28, 30, 31], although no effect has also been reported [42, 58]. Therefore, discrepancies regarding the variable responses to various doses of alcohol might be due to the different strains of rats used in the reported studies.

Behavioral responses may also be affected by other factors, including the light-dark cycle and the presence of stressful stimuli [52, 53]. Stimulant actions of alcohol on locomotor activity have been reported in rats in both normal and reverse light-dark cycles, although most studies have been carried out in normal cycle. For instance, alcohol at doses of 0.25 and 0.5 g/kg increased locomotor activity in FRL and Nijmegen Wistar rats, respectively [11, 28], whereas no effect was observed with alcohol doses of 0.1 – 0.5 g/kg in Sprague-Dawley, P, NP, FH and FSL rats [11, 42, 58]. On the other hand, alcohol-induced increases in horizontal activity with doses of 0.1 and 0.25 g/kg have been reported in Sprague-Dawley rats in reverse light-dark cycle [30, 43]. We have shown that a higher dose of alcohol (1 g/kg) also stimulates locomotor activity in non-selected Wistar rats in a reverse light-dark cycle. Thus, lower doses of alcohol are required to induce locomotor activity in Sprague-Dawley than in non-selected Wistar rats, suggesting the existence of differences in sensitivity to alcohol effects between different strains of rodents, as described by other authors [9, 10, 65, 66]. Moreover, alcohol low doses do not stimulate locomotor activity in Sprague-Dawley rats maintained in a normal cycle, while these doses elicit activating responses in reverse cycle animals. These findings indicate that behavioral responses to low doses of alcohol in the same rat strain are altered depending on the light-dark cycle.

In the present study we investigated the effects of alcohol in non-selected Wistar rats in reverse cycle, since motor activity was higher than that in normal cycle animals. However, a higher motor activity does not necessarily predict a higher alcohol stimulant effect. To our knowledge, the effects of different doses of alcohol have not been compared in both normal and reverse light-dark cycles in the same rat strain. Therefore, it would be interesting to determine if the alcohol stimulant actions observed in the present study are similar in both light-dark cycles.

Numerous studies have consistently shown that alcohol high doses (more than 2 g/kg) produce depressant effects in rodents [28, 31, 58, 62]. Accordingly, we have shown that an alcohol dose of 2.5 g/kg significantly decreased horizontal and stereotyped movements. These findings suggest that motor responses to high doses of alcohol may not be related to the rodent strain or the light-dark cycle and may be associated to the sedative effects of the drug.

Animal exposure to a certain stressful stimuli, such as a novel environment, triggers specific neural changes which determine behavioral responses to drugs of abuse. The environmental context in which drugs are administered modulates their ability to induce forms of drug experience-dependent plasticity [3, 12]. Behavioral responses to drugs, as well as gene expression patterns in specific brain regions are differentially modulated by the exposure to a novel environment [4, 13, 22, 23, 32, 54, 60, 61]. In addition, animals exhibit different responses to drugs depending on how they respond to a novel environment. Animals showing high motor activity in a novel environment (High Responders, HR) are more susceptible to self-administrate drugs than animals exhibiting low activity (Low Responders, LR) [8, 48]. These responses have been observed with amphetamine [48], dexamphetamine [20] and morphine [1]. Studies with alcohol have provided inconsistent results. Several reports have shown that spontaneous locomotor activity during a single exposure to a novel environment failed to predict alcohol intake [5, 38, 44]. In contrast, Gingras and Cools (1995) [27] found an inverse correlation between exposure to novelty and alcohol intake in Nijmegen Wistar rats, HR animals showing a significantly less alcohol intake than LR animals. Interestingly, the i.p. administration of alcohol doses of 0.25 and 0.5 g/kg stimulated locomotor activity in HR but not in LR animals [28, 30], suggesting that a novel stimulus predicts alcohol sensitivity in these animals. In contrast, high alcohol doses (i.e., 2 g/kg) produced sedative effects in both types of animals [28], indicating that depressant effects of alcohol are not altered by a novel stimulus. Therefore, alcohol stimulant and depressant actions on motor activity may involve different neural mechanisms. The behavioral response to an alcohol dose of 1 g/kg observed in the present study is worth mentioning, since this dose significantly increased horizontal and stereotyped movements, despite the fact that animals were not selected as High (HR) and Low (LR) responders. Research is currently carried out in our laboratory in order to study the dose-dependent actions of alcohol on locomotor activity in animals selected by their response to a novel stimulus.

Dopaminergic neurotransmission in the nucleus accumbens and the caudate-putamen plays a critical role in the mechanisms underlying the locomotor and stereotyped responses elicited by psychostimulant drugs, respectively [14, 33, 49, 59]. On the other hand, alcohol modulates the activity of dopaminergic reinforcement and reward circuits (i.e., the mesocortical and meso-accumbens systems) [34, 35, 36, 63], as well as the nigrostriatal pathway [66]. Regulation of dopaminergic transmission in these pathways plays a major role in controlling motor activity in response to alcohol exposure [39, 42, 62, 64]. Studies regarding the behavioral actions of alcohol have been mainly focused on horizontal activity [11, 28]. A few reports have assessed the effects of the drug on vertical activity [43], whereas the stereotyped movements induced by alcohol have been poorly investigated. We have shown that total horizontal activity and total stereotyped movements were significantly affected by alcohol administration at doses of 1g/kg and 2.5 g/kg : an alcohol dose of 1 g/kg increased, while a dose of 2.5 g/kg diminished both parameters. The locomotor and stereotyped responses induced by these alcohol doses might be related to dopaminergic activation in the nucleus accumbens and the caudate-putamen, respectively, as suggested by other authors for psychostimulants [14, 33, 49, 59]. Further research is needed in order to elucidate the mechanisms of action of alcohol in these brain circuits.

CONCLUSION

Behavioral responses to alcohol exposure are affected by several factors, including the dose and route of administration, the rodent strain, the light-dark cycle and the presence of stressful stimuli, such as a novel environment. In this study we have shown that non-selected Wistar rats in a reverse light-dark cycle exhibited a higher motor activity than animals in normal cycle. Alcohol administration in reverse cycle animals produced stimulant and depressant effects depending on the dose. An alcohol dose of 1 g/kg increased total horizontal activity and total stereotyped movements, while a dose of 2.5 g/kg showed opposite effects. Our results suggest that stimulant alcohol effects may be mainly attributed to fast horizontal and fast stereotyped movements. In contrast, the sedative alcohol effects may involve similar contributions of fast and slow horizontal, as well as fast stereotyped movements. Alcohol behavioral responses might be closely related to activation of brain dopaminergic circuits in the nucleus accumbens and the caudate-putamen.

ACKNOWLEDGMENTS

We thank Dr. L. Mayagoitia for helpful discussions and J.M. Luna and S. Rodriguez for technical assistance. This work was supported by Consejo Nacional de Ciencia y Tecnología (CONACyT) (34359-N and 42095-M).

REFERENCES

[1] Ambrosio, E., Goldberg S. R. and Elmer, G. I. (1995). Behavior genetic investigation of the relationship between spontaneous locomotor activity and the acquisition of morphine self-administration behavior. *Behav Pharmacol 6*, 229-237.

[2] Antelman, S. M., Eichler, A. J., Black, C. A. and Kocan, D. (1980). Interchangeability of stress and amphetamine in sensitization. *Science 207*, 329-331.

[3] Badiani, A., Browman, K. E. and Robinson, T. E. (1995). Influence of novel versus home environments on sensitization to the psychomotor stimulant effects of cocaine and amphetamine. *Brain Res 674*, 291-298.

[4] Badiani, A., Oates, M. M., Day, H. E. W., Watson, S. J., Akil, H. and Robinson, T. E. (1999). Environmental modulation of amphetamine-induced c-fos expression in D_1 versus D_2 striatal neurons. *Behav Brain Res 103*, 203-209.

[5] Bisaga, A. and Kostowski, W. (1993). Individual behavioral differences and ethanol consumption in Wistar rats. *Physiol Behav 54*, 1225-1131.

[6] Carlsson, A., Engel, J. and Svensson, T. H. (1972). Inhibition of ethanol induced excitation in mice and rats by alpha-methyl-p-tyrosine. *Psychopharmacologia 26*, 307-312.

[7] Chen, H. T., Casanova, M. F., Kleinman, J. E., Zito, M., Goldman, D. and Linnoila, M. (1991). ^{3}H-Paroxetine binding in brains of alcoholics. *Psychiatry Res 38*, 293-299.

[8] Cools, A. R. and Gingras, M.A. (1997). Nijmegen high and low responders to novelty: A new tool in the search after the neurobiology of drug abuse liability. *Pharmacol Biochem Behav 60*, 151-159.

[9] Crabbe, J. C., Kosobud, A., Young, E. R., Tam, B. R. and McSwigan, J. D. (1985). Bidirectional selection for susceptibility to ethanol withdrawal seizures in *mus musculus. Behav Genet 15*, 521-536.

[10] Crabbe, J. C., Feller, D. J., Terdal, E. S. and Merril C. D. (1990). Genetic compounds of ethanol response. *Alcohol 7*, 245-248.

[11] Criswell, H. E., Overstreet, D. H., Rezvani, A. H., Johnson, K. B., Simson, P. E., Knapp, D. J., Moy, S. S. and Breese, G. R. (1994). Effects of ethanol, MK-801, and chlordiazapoxide on locomotor stimulation from ethanol preference. *Alcohol Clin Exp Res 18*, 917-923.

[12] Crombag, H.S., Badiani, A. and Robinson, T. E. (1996). Signalled versus unsignalled intravenous amphetamine: large differences in the acute psychomotor response and sensitization. *Brain Res 722*, 227-231.

[13] Day, H. E. W., Badiani, A., Uslaner, J. M., Oates, M. M., Vittoz, N. M., Robinson T. E., Watson, S. J. Jr. and Akil, H. (2001). Environmental novelty differentially affects c-fos mRNA expression induced by amphetamine or cocaine in subregions of the bed nucleus of the stria terminalis and amygdala. *J Neurisc 21*, 732-740.

[14] Delfs, J. M., Schreiber, L. and Kelley, A. E. (1990). Microinjection of cocaine into the nucleus accumbens elicits locomotor activation in the rat. *J Neurosci 10,* 303-310.

[15] de Wit, H., Uhlenhuth, E. H. and Johanson, C. E. (1987). Individual differences in behavioral and subjective responses to alcohol. *Alcohol Clin Exp Res 11*, 52-59.

[16] de Wit, H., Pierri, J., Johanson, C. E. (1989). Assessing individual differences in ethanol preference using a cumulative dosing procedure. *Psychopharmacology 98*, 113-119.

[17] Duncan, P. M. and Baez, A. M. (1981). The effect of ethanol on wheel running in rats. *Pharmacol Biochem Behav 15,* 819-821.

[18] Earleywine, M. (1994). Anticipated biphasic effects of ethanol's psychomotor stimulant effect. *Alcohol Clin Exp Res 18,* 956-963.

[19] Erickson, C. K. and Kochhar, B. S. (1985). An animal model for low dose ethanol-induced locomotor stimulation: behavioral characteristics. *Alcohol Clin Exp Res 9,* 310-314.

[20] Exner, E. and Clark, D. (1993). Behavior in the novel environment predicts responsiveness to d-amphetamine in the rat: A multivariate approach. *Behav Pharmacol 4,* 47-56.

[21] Fadda, F., Argiolas, A., Melis, M. R., Serra, G. and Gessa, G. L. (1980). Differential effects of acute and chronic ethanol on dopamine metabolism in frontal cortex, caudate nucleus and substancia nigra. *Life Sci 27,* 979-986.

[22] Ferguson, S. M., Norton, C. S., Watson, S. J., Akil, H. and Robinson T. E. (2003). Amphetamine-evoked c-fos mRNA expression in the caudate-putamen: the effects of DA and NMDA receptor antagonists vary as a function of neuronal phenotype and environmental context. *J Neurochem 86,* 33-44.

[23] Ferguson, S. M. and Robinson, T. E. (2004). Amphetamine-evoked gene expression in striatopallidal neurons: regulation by corticostriatal afferents and the ERK/MAPK. *J Neurochem 91,* 337-348.

[24] Gauvin, D. V, Baird, T. J., Vanecek, S. A., Briscoe, R. J., Ballet, M. and Holloway, F. A. (1997). Effects of time-day and photoperiod phase shifts on voluntary ethanol consumption in rats. *Alcohol Clin Exp Res 21,* 817-825.

[25] Geller, I. (1971). Ethanol preference in the rat as a function of photoperiod. *Science 173,* 456-459.

[26] Gianoulakis, C. (1998). Alcohol-seeking behavior. *Alcohol Health Res World 27,* 202-210.

[27] Gingras, M. A. and Cools, A. R. (1995). Differential ethanol intake in high and low responders to novelty. *Behav Pharmacol 6,* 718-723.

[28] Gingras, M. A. and Cools, A. R. (1996). Analysis of the biphasic locomotor response to ethanol in high and low responders to novelty: a study in Nijmegen wistar rats. *Psychopharmacology 125,* 258-264.

[29] Grant, K. A. and Colombo, G. (1993). Discriminative stimulus effects of ethanol. Effect of training dose on the substitution of N-methyl-D-aspartate antagonists. *J Pharmacol Exp Ther 264*, 1241-1247.

[30] Hoshaw, B. A. and Lewis, M. J. (2001). Behavioral sensitization to ethanol in rats: Evidence from the Sprague-Dawley strain. *Pharmacol Biochem Behav 68*, 685-90.

[31] Imperato, A. and di Chiara, G. (1986). Preferential stimulation of dopamine release in the nucleus accumbens of freely moving rats. *J Pharmacol Exp Ther 239*, 219-228.

[32] Jaber, M., Cador, M., Dumartin, B., Normand, E., Stinus, L. and Bloch, B. (1995). Acute and chronic amphetamine treatments differently regulate neuropeptide messenger RNA levels and Fos immunoreactivity in rat striatal neurons. *Neuroscience 65*, 1041-1050.

[33] Kelly, P. H., Seviour, P. W. and Iversen, S. D. (1975). Amphetamine and apomorphine response in the rat following 6-OHDA lesions of the nucleus accumbens septi and corpus striatum. *Brain Res 94*, 507-522.

[34] Koob, G.F. (1992). Neural mechanisms of drug reinforcement. *Ann NY Acad Sci 654*, 171-191.

[35] Koob, G. F. (2003). Neuroadaptive mechanisms of addiction: studies on the extended amygdala. *Eur Neuropsychopharmacol 13*, 442-52.

[36] Koob, G. F., Ahmed, S. H., Boutrel, B., Chen, S. A., Kenny, P. J., Markou, A., O'Dell, L. E., Parsons, L. H. And Sanna, P. P. (2004). Neurobiological mechanisms in the transition from drug use to drug dependence. *Neurosci Biobehav Rev 27*, 739-49.

[37] Koros, E., Piasecki, J., Kostowski, W. and Bienkowski, P. (1998). Saccharin drinking rather than open field behavior predicts initial ethanol acceptance in Wistar rats. *Alcohol Alcohol 33*, 131-40.

[38] Koros, E., Plasecki, J., Kostowski, W. and Bienkowski, P. (1999). Development of alcohol deprivation effect in rats: lack of correlation with saccharin drinking and locomotor activity. *Alcohol Alcohol 34*, 542-50.

[39] Krimmer, E. C. and Schechter, M. D. (1992). HAD and LAD rats respond differently to stimulating effect but not discriminative effects of ethanol. *Alcohol 9*, 71-74.

[40] Lê, A. D., Quan, B., Juzytch, W., Fletcher, P. J., Joharchi, N. and Shaham, Y. (1998). Reinstatement of alcohol-seeking by priming injections of alcohol and exposure to stress in rats. *Psychopharmacology 135*, 169-174.

[41] Martin, C. S., Earleywine, M., Musty, R. E., Perrine, M. W. and Swift, R. M. (1993). Development and validation of the biphasic alcohol effects scale. *Alcohol Clin Exp Res 17*, 140-146.

[42] Milton, G. V., Patrick, K. and Erickson C. K. (1995). Low dose effects of ethanol on locomotor activity induced by activation of the Mesolimbic System. *Alcohol Clin Exp Res 19*, 3, 768-776.

[43] Moore, T. O., June, H. L. and Lewis, M. J. (1993). Ethanol induced stimulation and depression on measures of locomotor activity: effects of basal activity levels in rats. *Alcohol 10*, 537-40.

[44] Nadal, R. A., Pallares, M. A. and Ferre, N. S. (1996). Oral intake of sweetened or sweetened alcoholic beverages and open field behavior. *Pharmacol Biochem Behav 54*, 739-743.

[45] Nestby, P., Vanderschuren, L. J., de Vries, T. J., Hogenboom, F., Wardeh, G., Mulder, A. H. and Schoffelmeer, A. N. (1997). Ethanol, like psychostimulants and morphine,

causes long-lasting hyperreactivity of dopamine and acetylcholine neurons of rats nucleus accumbens: possible role in behavioral sensitization. *Psychopharmacology 133*, 69-76.

[46]   Oscar-Berman, M., Shagrin, B., Evert, D. L. and Epstein, C. (1997). Impairments of Brain and Behavior. *Alcohol Health Res World 21*, 65-75.

[47]   Phillips, T. J. and Shen, E. H. (1996). Neurochemical basis of locomotion and ethanol stimulant effects. *Int Rev Neurobiol 39*, 243-82

[48]   Piazza, P. V., Deminière, J. M., Maccari, S., Mormède, P., Le Moal, M. and Simon, H. (1990). Individual reactivity to novelty predicts probability of amphetamine self-administration. *Behav Pharmacol 1*, 339-345.

[49]   Pijnenburg, A. J. J., Honing, W. M. M. and Van Rossum J. M. (1975). Inhibition of the d-amphetamine-induced locomotor activity by injection of haloperidol into the nucleus accumbens of the rat. *Psychopharmacologia 41*, 87-95.

[50]   Pohorecky, L. A. (1991). Stress and alcohol interactions: An update of human research. *Alcoholism Clin Exp Res 15*, 438-58.

[51]   Reinberg, A. (1992). Circadian changes in psychologic effects of ethanol. *Neuropsychopharmacology 7*, 149-56.

[52]   Rosario, L. A. and Abercrombie, E. D. (1999). Individual differences in behavioral reactivity: correlation with stress-induced norepinephrine eflux in the hippocampus of Sprague-Dawley rats. *Brain Res Bull 48*, 595-602.

[53]   Rosenwasseer A.M. (2001) Alcohol, antidepresants, and Circadian Rhythms. *Alcohol Research and Health 25*, 126-135.

[54]   Ruskin, D. N., and Marshall, J. F. (1994). Amphetamine- and cocaine-induced fos in the rat striatum depends on D2 dopamine receptor activation. *Synapse 18*, 233-240.

[55]   Russell, V. A., Lamm, M .C. L. and Taljaard, J. J. F. (1988). Effect of ethanol on (^{3}H) dopamine release in rat nucleus accumbens and striatal slices. *Neurochemical Res 13*, 487-92.

[56]   Rybkin, I. I., Zhou, Y., Volaufova, J., Smagin, G. N., Ryan, D. H. and Harris, R. B. (1997). Effect of restraint stress on food intake and body weight is determined by time of day. *Am J Physiol 273*, 1612-1622.

[57]   Samson, H. H., Haraguchi, M., Tolliver, G. A. and Sadeghi, K. G. (1989). Antagonism of ethanol-reinforced behavior by the benzodiazepine inverse agonist Ro 15-4513 and FG 7142: relation to sucrose reinforcement. *Pharmacol Biochem Behav 33*, 601-608.

[58]   Schaeffer, G. J., Richardson, W. R., Bonsall, R. W. and Michael, R. P. (1988). Brain self-stimulation, locomotor activity and tissue concentrations of ethanol in male rats. *Drug Alcohol Depend 21*, 67-75.

[59]   Sharp, T., Zetterström T., Ljungberg T., Ungerstedt U. (1987). A direct comparison of amphetamine-induced behaviors and regional brain dopamine release in the rat using intracerebral microdialysis. *Brain Res 401*, 322-330.

[60]   Uslaner, J., Badin, A., Norton, C. S., Day, H. E. W., Watson, S. J., Akil, H. and Robinson, T. E. (2001). Amphetamine and cocaine induce different patterns of *c-fos* mRNA expression in the striatum and subthalamic nucleus depending on environmental context. Eur J *Neurosci 13*, 1977-1983.

[61]   Uslaner, J. M., Norton, C. S., Watson, S. J., Akil, H., and Robinson, E. (2003). Amphetamine-induced *c-fos* mRNA expression in the caudate-putamen and

subthalamic nucleus: interactions between dose, environment and neuronal phenotype. *J Neurochem 85*, 105-114.

[62] Waller, M. B., Murphy, J. M., McBride, W. J., Lumeng, L. and Li, T. K. (1986). Effect of low-dose ethanol on spontaneous motor activity in alcohol-preferring and non-preferring lines of rats. *Pharmacol Biochem Behav 24*, 617-623.

[63] Wise R. A. and Bozarth, M. A. (1982). Action of drugs of abuse on brain reward systems: an update with specific attention to opiates. *Pharmacol Biochem Behav 17*, 239-243.

[64] Wise R. A. and Bozarth, M. A. (1987). A psychomotor stimulant theory of addiction. *Psychol Rev 94*, 469-492.

[65] Yanai, J., Bergman, A., Keltz, M. and Pick, C. G. Mechanism of sensitivity and tolerance to ethanol and barbiturates. In: Yanai, J., Rosenfeld, J.M., Eldar, P. and Bauml, R. Alcohol dependence, the family and the community. London: Freund; 1988; pp. 143-158.

[66] Yanai, J., Shaanani, R. and Pick, C. G. (1995). Altered brain sensitivity to ethanol in mice after MPTP treatment. *Alcohol 12*, 127-30.

In: New Trends in Brain Research
Editor: F. J. Chen, pp. 143-157

ISBN 1-59454-834-X
© 2006 Nova Science Publishers, Inc.

Chapter VII

NEURONAL CYCLOOXYGENASE-2, MCL-1, BCL-X$_S$, BAX, CASPASE-6 AND −8 ACCUMULATION IN BRAINS OF PATIENTS WITH CREUTZFELDT-JAKOB DISEASE: FRIEND OR FOE?

Martin H. Deininger[1] and Richard Meyermann[*][2]
[1] Department of Neurosurgery, University of Freiburg Medical School,
Freiburg, Germany
[2] Institute of Brain Research, University of Tuebingen Medical School,
Tuebingen, Germany

ABSTRACT

Neuronal apoptosis in Creutzfeldt-Jakob disease (CJD) is well documented. However, little is known about associated signaling pathways. Recent results have demonstrated close interactions of cyclooxygenases, BCL-2 family members and caspases in the regulation of survival of central nervous system cells including neurons and their involvement in the modulation of apoptosis in diseases of the brain. Their localization in brains of CJD patients, however, remains unresolved.

We have now used immunocytochemistry to analyze expression of BCL-2, MCL-1, BCL-X$_S$, BAX and BAD of the BCL-2 family of proteins and of caspase-1, -2$_L$, -3, 6, -8 and -9 of the caspase family in frontal cortex slices of eight postmortem brains of sporadic CJD patients and three neuropathologically unaltered controls. Double labeling experiments confirmed the neuronal origin of BCL-2 and caspase family expressing cells. We observed accumulation of antiapoptotic MCL-1 (P= 0.004), proapoptotic BCL-X$_S$ (P=0.016) and BAX (P=0.016) and of caspase-6 (P<0.001) and −8 (P<0.001) in cortical

[*] Corresponding author: Department of Neurosurgery, University of Freiburg Medical School, Breisacher Str. 64, D-79106 Freiburg, Germany, Tel: +49-761-270-5001, FAX: +49-761-270-5090, Email: martin.deininger@uni-tuebingen.de

neurons of CJD compared to controls. Immunoreactivity of the other analyzed BCL-2 and caspase family members was only rarely observed in singular neurons in both, CJD patients and controls. Abundant data has previously demonstrated that effectors of cyclooxygenases, nonsteroidal anti-inflammatory drugs, induce the alteration of BCL-2 and caspase family members to influence cellular survival. Cyclooxygenases (COX) mediate inflammation, immunomodulation, blood flow, apoptosis and fever in various diseases of the brain. While COX-2 is cytokine-inducible, COX-1 is expressed by macrophages/microglial cells that accumulate in pathological foci. In a previous report, we observed significant accumulation of COX-1 in macrophages/microglial cells adjacent to neurons in brains of patients with Creutzfeldt-Jakob disease. COX-2 was predominantly observed in neurons, and their number was significantly higher compared to controls.

Although formal proof is lacking, our data therefore may indicate that NSAIDs may influence the course of CJD. However, the cyclooxygenase-BCL-2 family-caspase pathway is a modulator not only of apoptosis, but also of cellular differentiation, immune-reaction and angiogenesis. Therefore, additional data needs to be acquired to justify clinical trials using NSAIDs in these patients.

Key words: Apoptosis - BCL-2 family – Cyclooxygenase-1 – Cyclooxygenase-2 - Caspase family - Creutzfeldt-Jakob disease

INTRODUCTION

Clinical and pathological descriptions of what is now referred to as Creutzfeldt-Jakob disease (CJD) first appeared in the early 1920s. Over subsequent years, a number of similar conditions were described with a variety of eponyms. It was not until 1968, however, when the direct experimental transmission of CJD from a human to a chimpanzee was first reported, that the existence of a unique disease entity was fully established and the term "Creutzfeldt-Jakob disease" was universally accepted [1,2]. Since then, CJD has been recognized in both sporadic and familial forms, and its unintentional transmission from one human to another (iatrogenic CJD) has been tragically documented, mainly through the use of cadaveric human growth hormone or dura mater grafts manufactured before the mid-1980s [3-5]. Still, CJD remained a fairly obscure form of dementia until recent years. It has now achieved broader notoriety in the wake of extensive media coverage of another prion disease, bovine spongiform encephalopathy (BSE), commonly referred to as "mad cow disease," and its probable transmission to humans in the United Kingdom [6].

Human transmissible spongiform encephalopathies (TSEs) or prion diseases are neurodegenerative disorders of infectious, inherited or sporadic origin and include Creutzfeldt-Jakob disease (CJD), Gerstmann-Straussler-Scheinker disease (GSS), kuru and fatal familial insomnia (FFI) [7]. A recent report has revealed that prominent neuronal apoptosis can be observed in CJD patients independent of the origin of the disease, familial, sporadic or iatrogenic, suggesting common downstream alterations in neuronal degeneration of patients with TSE [8]. Furthermore, a rodent model of TSE confirmed increased numbers of apoptotic neurons in scrapie infected mice [9] and the 106-126 synthetic peptide homologous to prion protein (PrP) has shown to be neurotoxic and induce apoptosis in rat hippocampal neurons in vitro [10].

In degenerative brain disease, the BCL-2 and caspase protein families are well known modulators of neuronal apoptosis. While the BCL-2 family of proteins initiates apoptosis, caspases are regarded as downstream mediators of BCL-2 induction. Close interactions of both protein families are a well known consequence. BCL-2 family proteins are proto-oncogenes that determine apoptotic cell death and proliferation in a wide range of human neoplasms. Thus, both antiapoptotic gene products such as BCL-2, BCL-X and MCL-1, and proapoptotic gene products such as BAX are differentially expressed in patients with degenerative brain disease and might contribute to short survival and early progression [11]. Up- or down-regulation of single members of the BCL-2 family alter the overall susceptibility to apoptosis in mammalian cells. BCL-2 has been shown to block apoptosis [12-14]. Two distinct BCL-X mRNAs are generated by alternative splicing. BCL-XL inhibits cell death, similar to BCL-2, whereas the short variant, BCL-XS, inhibits the ability of BCL-2 to block cell death [15]. The expression of MCL-1, another antiapoptotic BCL-2 family protein [16], increases rapidly in response to differentiation-inducing agents and in response to colchicine and vinblastine. Therefore, MCL-1 may serve as a modulator of cell viability that can undergo rapid up-regulation as well as down-regulation, with up-regulation associated with differentiation or death [17]. BAX has extensive amino acid homology with BCL-2. BAX accelerates apoptotic death induced by cytokine deprivation and counters the death repressor activity of BCL-2. The ratio of BCL-2 to BAX may therefore determine survival or death in response to an apoptotic stimulus [18]. The biological function of BCL-2 proteins is determined by complex dimerization patterns with each other and with proteins unrelated to BCL-2 at binding sites termed BH1, BH2 and BH3 [19]. Binding of pro-apoptotic members of the BCL-2 family constitutes a distinct mechanism of cell protection from apoptosis [20]. The binding of BH3-containing proteins such as Bad promotes cell death by binding to antiapoptotic members of the BCL-2 family and thus inhibiting their survival-promoting functions [21]. However, mechanisms other than dimerization among members of the BCL-2 family are probably involved in the regulation of apoptosis by these proteins [22]: BCL-2 family members bind to nonhomologous proteins and are capable to form ion channels and pores [23].

Cysteine aspartate-specific proteases (caspases) are the proteases that are responsible for the systematic dismantling of a cell commited to die [24]. The caspase family of apoptosis modulators are cysteine proteases which have the capacity to cleave aspartic acid residues and form three subfamilies. Prodomains of the initiator caspases (caspase-2, -8, -9, -10) contain caspase recruitment domains that have a regulatory role by serving to couple cellular signaling pathways to caspase activation [24-26]. Activator initiator caspases then cleave and acitvate effector caspases (caspase-3, -6, -7). In turn, cleave cellular substrates. The last group of caspases (caspase-1, -4, -5, -11, -12, -13, -14) are inflammatory caspases that extend the involvement of caspases to inflammatory diseases [27]. However, only caspases-1, -2, -3, -6, -8 and –9 have been associated with Alzheimer´s disease in particular that shares considerable similarities with CJD in pathophysiological mechanisms.

Cyclooxygenases (COX, prostaglandin endoperoxide synthases, PGH synthases) catalyze the synthesis of the eicosanoid prostaglandin metabolites PGG_2 and PGH_2 which are metabolized to PGE_2, PGD_2 and $PGF_{2\alpha}$, the thromboxane TXA_2, or the functional antagonist of TXA_2, PGI_2 (prostacyclin). Eicosanoids are differential regulators of blood perfusion.

PGE$_2$ and PGE$_1$ are powerful dilators of the vasculature that result in a decrease of the peripheral resistance and a consequent decrease of blood pressure. Inversely, PGF$_{2\alpha}$ increases the blood pressure. Apart from affecting the cardiovascular system, differential eicosanoid effects can be observed in the hematopoietic system and a broad range of organs like the kidney, smooth muscle and the gut. Further, eicosanoids are potential modulators of the immune system. PGs of the E series mediate the liberation of histamin from mast cells during anaphylaxy, inhibit the liberation of oxygen radicals from activated leukocytes, the differentiation of B cells and the proliferation of T cells. Macrophage-derived PGE$_2$ has been shown to inhibit the liberation of lymphokines from activated T cells.

Two COX isoforms have been described [28]. While COX-1 is an enzyme of a molecular mass of 66 kd that is constitutively expressed in a range of tissues, COX-2 is a 70 kd interferon gamma (IFN-γ)-inducible homologue that shares 61% sequence identity with COX-1. The expression of COX-1 and COX-2 has been reported to be associated with the complex derangements observed during a variety of diseases of the brain. Following trauma, prostaglandins cause vascular damage [29]. Cerebral ischemia leads to upregulation of COX-2 message, protein, and reaction products in the injured hemispheres [30]. For years, inhibition of cyclooxygenase was regarded as a novel therapy strategy to treat patients with degenerativ brain disease [31]. However, a recent report showed detrimental effects of cyclooxygenase inhibition, thus shedding new light on the subject [32].

In order to reveal the involvement of BCL-2 and caspase family members in CJD patients and thus provide evidence for a new rationale in treating theses patients, we have used immunocytochemistry to analyze expression of BCL-2, MCL-1, BCL-X$_S$, BAX and BAD of the BCL-2 family of proteins and caspase-1, -2$_L$, -3, 6, -8 and -9 of the caspase family of proteins in postmortem brains of eight sporadic CJD and three neuropathologically unaltered control patients.

PATIENTS AND METHODS

Patients

Frontal cortex slices of brains of eight patients who died of sporadic Creutzfeldt-Jakob disease and of three neuropathologically unaltered control patients were analyzed (Table 1). All CJD brains examined exhibited the typical CJD histopathology as confirmed by routine diagnosis of two independent neuropathologists. Prior death, CJD and control patients who suffered severe heart attacs or lung embolism were treated and diagnosed in other departments of the Tuebingen University clinics. Other diseases (neoplasia, infection, degeneration or additction) were excluded by routine diagnosis. All brains were removed and diagnosed at the Institute of Brain Research according to the ethical guidelines for routine pathological examination in Tuebingen and have in part been characterized before [33]]. Postmortem times ranged from few hours to one day and did not differ significantly between the patients.

Table 1. Immunohistochemical labeling scores of BCL-2 family proteins in Creutzfeldt-Jakob disease and control patients

Entry #	Gender /age	Diagnosis	BCL-2	MCL-1	BCL-X$_S$	BAX	BAD	C1	C2	C3	C6	C8	C9
ES 230/98	M /31	normal	0	0	1	1	0	1	0	0	0	1	0
ES 220/95	M /25	normal	0	1	1	1	1	1	0	1	0	1	1
ES 200/97	F / 82	normal	2	1	1	1	0	1	0	1	0	1	1
ES 190/00	M /79	CJD	0	3	3	3	1	1	0	1	3	3	0
ES 27/94	F / 74	CJD	0	4	3	3	1	3	1	1	3	3	1
ES 209/93	F / 80	CJD	0	3	3	2	0	2	1	1	3	3	1
ES 79/93	M / 56	CJD	1	3	1	1	0	3	1	2	3	3	1
ES 68/93	F / 81	CJD	1	4	3	3	0	0	1	1	3	4	1
ES 222/96	M / 80	CJD	1	4	3	3	3	2	2	1	3	3	1
ES 284/91	M / 56	CJD	0	3	3	3	0	0	1	1	2	3	3
ES 51/94	F / 75	CJD	1	4	2	3	0	0	1	0	2	3	1

Labeling score was determined 0= no labeled cells, 1= up to 5% labeled cells, 2= 6% - 20% labeled cells, 3= 21% - 50% labeled cells, 4= more than 51% labeled cells. M = male, F = female, C=Caspase. Patient age is shown in years.

Immunohistochemistry

Tissues were pretreated with formic acid and buffered 4% formalin to be embedded in paraffin by routine methods. Fixation times ranged from one to three days. Five μm sections of the neocortex were cut, deparaffinized and rehydrated. For antigen retrieval, the sections were immersed in 0.01 M citrate buffer and irradiated in a microwave oven set at 750 W, five cycles of 5 min. Endogenous peroxidase was blocked with 1% H_2O_2 in methanol and the slices were consequently incubated with porcine serum. Mouse monoclonal antibody directed against BCL-2 (clone 124, Dakopatts, Glostrup, Denmark) and rabbit polyclonal monospecific antibodies directed against MCL-1 (S19), BCL-X$_S$ (L19), BAX (P19) and BAD (C7) (all Santa Cruz, Santa Cruz, CA, USA) and previously descibed monospecific antibodies directed against caspase-1 (C-20), caspase-2$_L$ (C-20), caspase-6 (K-20), caspase-8 (T-16), caspase-9 (H-170, all Santa Cruz Biotech, Santa Cruz, CA, USA) and caspase-3 (New England Biolabs, Beverly, MA, USA) were diluted in Tris-buffered saline (TBS) and applied overnight at 4°C at the following concentrations: 1:1000 (L19, P19, C7), 1:500 (S19), 1:100

(124, caspase-1, -2_L, 3, 6, 8, 9) [34,35]. Biotinylated anti-mouse IgG (Dakopatts) or anti-rabbit IgG (Dakopatts) both diluted at 1:400 in TBS-BSA and streptavidin-biotin horseradish peroxidase complex (Dakopatts) diluted 1:400 were used for the detection of tissue-bound antibodies. Finally, diamenobenzidine (Sigma, St.Louis, MO) was used for visualization.

Double Labeling Experiments

In double labeling experiments, slices were deparaffinized, irradiated in a microwave oven for antigen retrieval and incubated with nonspecific porcine serum as described above. Then the differentiating antibodies directed against GFAP (glial fibrillary acidic protein, Boehringer Mannheim, Germany), HLA-DR, -DP, -DQ (MHC class II), CD68 (macrophages), CD3 (T-cells), CD20 (B-cells), vWF (von-Willebrand factor, endothelial cells), and NSE (Neuron-specific enolase) (all Dakopatts, Glostrup, Denmark) were added to the slices at a dilution of 1:100 in TBS-BSA. Visualization was achieved by adding biotinylated rabbit anti-mouse IgG or biotinylated swine anti-rabbit IgG, both diluted 1:400 in BSA-TBS for 30 min and alkaline phosphatase conjugated ABC complex diluted 1:400 in BSA-TBS for 30 min. Consecutively, we developed with Fast Blue BB salt chromogen-substrate solution yielding a blue reaction product. Between double labeling experiments, slices were irradiated in a microwave for 20 min in citrate buffer. Then BCL-2 family and caspase antibodies were immunolabeled as described above.

Evaluation and Controls

Adjacent sections were stained with irrelevant isotype-matched antibodies as controls. Immunoblot studies were described previously to confirm that the antibodies to the BCL-2 family proteins detected only one band of predicted size in glioma cell lines and were not mutually cross-reactive [35]. Single labeled sections were counterstained with hematoxylin. For evaluation, positively stained neurons were counted in 4 randomly chosen 200x magnification fields and compared to the total number of counterstained neurons using an eye-piece grid. Samples with no positive cells were classified as negative (0), samples with singular (up to 5%) positive cells as weakly positive (1), samples with 6-20 % positive cells as moderately positive (2), samples with 21% - 50% positive cells as strongly positive (3), and samples with more than 51% positive cells as very strongly positive (4). Mean labeling scores (MLS) were calculated and compared using the Mann-Whitney U-test.

RESULTS

BCL-2 Immunohistochemistry

BCL-2, MCL-1, BCL-X_S, BAX and BAD immunoreactivity in eight frontal cortical slices of postmortem brains of patients who died with CJD and three neuropathologically unaltered controls were analyzed by immunocytochemistry. In patients without neuropathological alterations, only singular disseminated neurons were labeled by BCL-2 (MLS = 0.66, SEM = 0.66, Figure 1A), MCL-1 (MLS = 0.66, SEM = 0.33, Figure 1C), BCL-X$_S$ (MLS = 1.03, SEM = 0.03, Figure 1E), BAX (MLS = 1.03, SEM = 0.03, Figure 1G) and BAD (MLS = 0.33, SEM = 0.33, Figure 1I), (Table 1). In patients who died with sporadic Creutzfeldt-Jakob disease, we observed significant accumulation of neurons labeled by MCL-1 (MLS = 3.5, SEM = 0.2; P=0.004; Figure 1D), BCL-X$_S$ (MLS = 2.6, SEM = 0.26; P=0.016; Figure 1F) and BAX (MLS = 2.6, SEM = 0.26; P=0.016; Figure 1H). Inversely, insignificant numbers of neurons expressed BCL-2 (MLS = 0.5, SEM = 0.2; P=0.57; Figure 1B) and BAD (MLS = 0.63, SEM = 0.38; P=0.68; Figure 1K) compared to controls. Double labeling experiments with antibodies directed against GFAP (glial cells), HLA-DR, -DP, -DQ (macrophages/microglial cells), CD68 (macrophages/microglial cells), CD3 (T-cells), CD20 (B-cells), vWF (von-Willebrand factor, endothelial cells), and NSE (neurons) were used to ensure that counted cells were of neuronal origin. Although the predominant cell type of BCL-2 family immunoreactivity were neurons, singular astrocytes and macrophages/microglial cells occasionally were occasionally labeled.

Caspase Immunohistochemistry

In patients without neuropathological alterations, only singular disseminated neurons were labeled by caspase-1 (MLS = 0.66, SEM = 0.33, Figure 2A), caspase-2 (MLS = 0.33, SEM = 0.33, Figure 2C), caspase-3 (MLS = 0.66, SEM = 0.33, Figure 2E), caspase-6 (MLS = 0.33, SEM = 0.33, Figure 2G), caspase-8 (MLS = 0.66, SEM = 0.33, Figure 2I) and caspase-9 (MLS = 0.66, SEM = 0.33, Figure 2L), (Table 1). In patients who died with sporadic Creutzfeldt-Jakob disease, we observed significant accumulation of neurons labeled by caspase-6 (MLS = 2.75, SEM = 0.16; P<0.001; Figure 2H) and caspase-8 (MLS = 3.13, SEM = 0.13; P<0.001; Figure 2K). Inversely, insignificant numbers of neurons and astrocytes or macrophages/microglial cells expressed caspase-1 (MLS=1.38, SEM= 0.46, Figure 2B), -2$_L$ (MLS=1.0, SEM= 0.19, Figure 2D), -3 (MLS=1.0, SEM= 0.19, Figure 2F) and −9 (MLS=1.13, SEM= 0.3, Figure 2M) compared to controls. Again, double labeling experiments showed that the counted cells were of neuronal origin. Only singular macrophages/microglial cells and a minority of astrocytes showed caspase immunoreactivity.

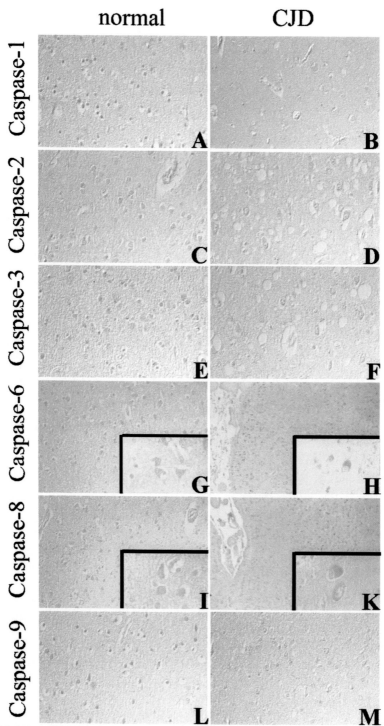

Figure 1. (A)-(K) Comparative BCL-2 family immunoreactivity (brown color) in CJD and control patients. A-K x400. All slices are counterstained with hematoxylin (blue color).

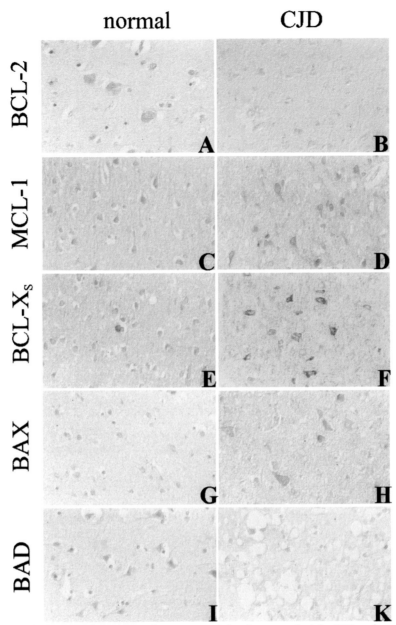

Figure 2. (A)-(M) Comparative caspase immunoreactivity (brown color) in CJD and control patients. A-F,L,M x200, G,H x40, inserts x1000. All slices are counterstained with hematoxylin (blue color).

DISCUSSION

CJD is considered a rare disease, however iatrogenic transmission might contribute to major epidemiological sequelae. Although neuronal loss is the predominant underlying mechanism of the observed clinical phenomena, little is known about upstream signaling cascades involved in this process.

Neuronal subsets of parvalbumin positive GABAergic inhibitory interneurons that are found in the frontal cortex have been recently demonstrated to be selectively vulnerable in neurodegenerative disorders such as TSEs, Alzheimer's disease, Parkinson's disease, Pick's disease, and others [1]. Although formal proof is lacking, some insight into these processes were drawn from experimental data. BCL-2 family proteins are differentially involved in this process. Among others, BAX-mediated apoptosis in neurons is involved in many pathologic conditions affecting the central nervous system, including degenerative diseases. Accumulation of proapoptotic BAX and BCL-X_S has been reported to participate in neuronal cell death [36,37]. Inversely, accumulation of antiapoptotic MCL-1 has not been described in brain disease [38]. In this context, it is of note that we observed significant accumulation of antiapoptotic MCL-1, proapoptotic BCL-X_S and BAX in cortical neurons of patients who died with CJD. These findings are of note, because MCL-1 preferentially binds to BAX to inhibit its proapoptotic function, but not to BCL- X_S. Therefore, our data might indicate that BCL- X_S overexpression in CJD patients in vivo appears to constitute a proapoptotic pathway that leads to increased neuronal cell death as previously shown in rat ischemia and other diseases of the brain [36].

We observed upregulation only of caspase-6 and –8 in neurons of CJD patients. While formal proof for the involvement of caspases in neuronal cell death in Creutzfeldt-Jakob disease patients is lacking, it is well documented in other diseases of the brain. Caspase-1 activation was observed in brains of patients and mice with Huntington´s disease and expression of a dominant-negative caspase-1 mutant extended survival and delayed the appearance of neuronal inclusions, neurotransmitter receptor alterations and onset of symptoms [39]. Increased amounts of caspase-1 were observed in Alzheimer´s disease [40] and in a range of in vitro systems of neuronal degeneration [41]. Caspase-2 has two messenger RNAs generated by alternative splicing, termed caspase-2L and caspase-2S. Although caspase-2L induces apoptosis, caspase-2S also has the ability to antagonize cell death. Caspase-2 mediates neuronal cell death induced by beta-amyloid [42] and induces apoptosis in a wide range of cell lines [43]. Caspase-3 is induced following traumatic axonal injury [44], induces apoptosis in Parkinson´s disease [45] and is involved in the developmental maturation of neurons [46]. Activated Caspase-9 cleaves downstream caspases such as Caspase-3, -6 and -7 initiating the caspase cascade. When cells receive apoptotic stimuli, mitochondria release cytochrome c which then binds to Apaf-1, the mammalian Ced-4 homologue, together with dATP. The resultant complex recruits Caspase-9 leading to its activation. In neuronal cell culture models, apoptosis-inducing agents trigger translocation of caspase-9 from mitochondria to the nucleus, which is inhibitable by Bcl-2. Similarly, in an animal model of transient global cerebral ischemia, caspase-9 release from mitochondria and accumulation in nuclei was observed in hippocampal and other vulnerable neurons exhibiting early postischemic changes preceding apoptosis [47].

Upregulation of caspase-6 and –8 has been described to be involved in neuronal degeneration before. In a model of Alzheimer´s disease, inhibition of caspase-6 activity prevents serum deprivation-mediated increase of Abeta. Caspase-6 directly cleaves APP at the C terminus and generates a C-terminal fragment of 3 kDa (Capp3) and an Abeta-containing 6.5-kDa fragment, Capp6.5, that increases in serum-deprived neurons. Caspase-6 proenzyme is present in adult human brain tissue, and the p10 active caspase-6 fragment is detected in AD brain tissue [48]. Caspase-8 causes beta-amyloid-induced apoptosis [49] and is expressed by different populations of cortical neurons undergoing delayed cell death after focal stroke in the rat [50]. Moreover, close interactions of caspase-8 and BAX have been described. Upregulation of both proteins is a well-known phenomenon and has been described in a wide variety of cell types [51]. Caspases are synthesized as zymogens and can be activated by cleavage, by oligomerization, or by interacting with an adapter molecule to form an apoptosome [51, 52]. Two different pathways of caspase activation leading to cell death have been identified, an intrinsic and an extrinsic pathway [53]. The intrinsic death pathway involves mitochondrial release of cytochrome c, which interacts with Apaf-1, an adapter protein, to form an apoptosome that activates caspase-9 [54]. The extrinsic pathway involves activation of death receptors, such as Fas, and recruitment of caspase-8 via interaction of adapter proteins with the receptor's death domain [53]. Caspase-8 then activates effector caspases, such as caspase-3, -6, and -7. Caspase-8 can also activate the intrinsic pathway by cleavage of BID, which induces mitochondrial release of cytochrome c [55].

Recent studies show close interactions of cyclooxygenases, caspase and BCL-2 family function. COX-2 inhibitors interfere with calcium signaling [56]. COX-2 inhibitors perturb intracellular Ca^{2+} by blocking endoplasmic reticulum Ca^{2+}-ATPases [57, 58]. The consequence of inhibiting this Ca^{2+} reuptake mechanism is Ca^{2+} mobilization from the endoplasmic reticulum stores and extracellular calcium influx leading to cytosolic Ca^{2+} elevation [59]. Sustained cytosolic Ca^{2+} elevation has been shown to impose adverse effects on the cell [60]. Mitochondrial uptake of excess cytosolic Ca^{2+} yields cytochrome c release and triggers apoptosis via caspase activation [60,61]. It has been suggested that COX-2 inhibitors exert their therapeutic activity through mechanisms that are independent of their COX-2 inhibitory activity [62]. Proposed non-COX cellular targets are AKT, IκB, and kinase ß, the peroxisome proliferator-activated receptor family of nuclear hormone receptors, and the proapoptotic gene Bax [63-65]

Accordingly, several studies conducted by other investigators have demonstrated that an inhibitor of cyclooxygenase-2, celecoxib, suppresses the proliferation of various cells by inducing apoptosis [66-71], suggesting that the proapoptotic action of celecoxib may be useful for the chemoprevention of tumorigenesis [68,70]. In degenerative brain alterations, however, these phenomena add to the destructive course of the disease [32].

Selective expression of MCL-1, BCL-X$_S$ and BAX and of caspase-6 and -8 in cortical neurons of patients who died with CJD therefore provides evidence for the involvement of apoptotic signaling cascades. The use of inhibitors of cyclooxygenases in theses patients, however, may have destructive consequences.

REFERENCES

[1]   Gibbs CJ Jr, Gajdusek DC, Asher DM, et al: Creutzfeldt-Jakob disease (spongiform encephalopathy): transmission to a chimpanzee. *Science* 161:388-389, 1968

[2]   Johnson RT, Gibbs CJ: Creutzfeldt-Jakob disease and related transmissible spongiform encephalopathies. *N Engl J Med* 339:1994-2004, 1998

[3]   Duffy P, Wolf J, Collins G, et al: Possible person-to-person transmission of Creutzfeldt-Jakob disease. *N Engl J Med* 290:692-693, 1974

[4]   Bernoulli C, Seigfried J, Baumgartner G, et al: Danger of accidental person-to-person transmission of Creutzfeldt-Jakob disease by surgery. *Lancet* 1:478-479, 1977

[5] Brown P, Preece M, Brandel J-P, et al: Iatrogenic Creutzfeldt-Jakob disease at the millennium. *Neurology* 55:1075-1081, 2001

[6] Bruce ME, Will RG, Ironside JW, et al: Transmissions to mice indicate that "new-variant" CJD is caused by the BSE agent. *Nature* 389:498-501, 1997

[7] Guentchev M, Wanschitz J, Voigtlander T, Flicker H, Budka H. Selective neuronal vulnerability in human prion diseases. Fatal familial insomnia differs from other types of prion diseases. *Am J Pathol* 1999;155:1453-7

[8] Gray F, Chretien F, Adle-Biassette H, Dorandeu A, Ereau T, Delisle MB, Kopp N, Ironside JW, Vital C. Neuronal apoptosis in Creutzfeldt-Jakob disease. *J Neuropathol Exp Neurol* 1999;58:321-8

[9] Giese A, Groschup MH, Hess B, Kretzschmar HA. Neuronal cell death in scrapie-infected mice is due to apoptosis. *Brain Pathol* 1995;5:213-21

[10] Forloni G, Angeretti N, Chiesa R, Monzani E, Salmona M, Bugiani O, Tagliavini F. Neurotoxicity of a prion protein fragment. *Nature* 1993;362:543-6

[11] Engidawork E, Gulesserian T, Seidl R, Cairns N, Lubec G. Expression of apoptosis related proteins in brains of patients with Alzheimer's disease. *Neurosci Lett* 2001 303;79-82.

[12] Hockenbery D, Nunez G, Milliman C, Schreiber RD, Korsmeyer SJ. Bcl-2 is an inner mitochondrial membrane protein that blocks programmed cell death. *Nature* 1990;348:334-6.

[13] Garcia I, Martinou I, Tsujimoto Y, Martinou JC. Prevention of programmed cell death of sympathetic neurons by the bcl-2 proto-oncogene. *Science* 1992;258:302-4.

[14] Weller M, Malipiero U, Aguzzi A, Reed JC, Fontana A. Protooncogene bcl-2 gene transfer abrogates Fas/APO-1 antibody-mediated apoptosis of human malignant glioma cells and confers resistance to chemotherapeutic drugs and therapeutic irradiation. *J Clin Invest* 1995;95:2633-43.

[15] Boise LH, Gonzales-Garcia M, Postema CE. Bcl-x, a Bcl-2 related gene that functions as a dominant regulator of apoptotic cell death. *Cell* 1993;71:557-560.

[16] Reynolds JE, Yang T, Qian L, Jenkinson JD, Zhou P, Eastman A, et al. MCL-1, a member of the Bcl-2 family, delays apoptosis induced by c-myc overexpression in chinese hamster ovary cells. *Cancer Res* 1994;54:6348-52.

[17] Yang T, Buchan HL, Townsend KJ, Craig RW. MCL-1, a member of the BLC-2 family, is induced rapidly in response to signals for cell differentiation or death, but not to signals for cell proliferation. *J Cell Physiol* 1996;166:523-36.

[18] Oltvai ZN, Milliman CL, Korsmeyer SJ. Bcl-2 heterodimerizes in vivo with a conserved homolog, Bax, that accelerates programmed cell death. *Cell* 1993;74:609-19.

[19] Yin XM, Oltvai ZN, Korsmeyer SJ. BH1 and BH2 domains of Bcl-2 are required for inhibition of apoptosis and heterodimerization with Bax. *Nature* 1994;369:321-3.

[20] Ottilie S, Diaz JL, Chang J, Wilson G, Tuffo KM, Weeks S, et al. Structural and functional complementation of an inactive Bcl-2 mutant by Bax truncation. *J Biol Chem* 1997;272:16955-61.

[21] Kelekar A, Chang BS, Harlan JE, Fesik SW, Thompson CB. Bad is a BH3 domain-containing protein that forms an inactivating dimer with Bcl-XL. *Mol Cell Biol* 1997;17:7040-6.

[22] Hsu YT, Youle RJ. Bax in murine thymus is a soluble monomeric protein that displays differential detergent-induced conformations. *J Biol Chem* 1998;273:10777-83.

[23] Schendel SL, Xie Z, Montal MO, Matsuyama S, Montal M, Reed JC. Channel formation by antiapoptotic protein Bcl-2. *Proc Natl Acad Sci* USA 1997;94:5113-8

[24] Thornberry NA, Lazebnik Y. Caspases: enemies within. *Science* 1998;281:1312-6

[25] Wolf BB, Green DR. Suicidal tendencies: apoptotic cell death by caspase family proteinases. *J Biol Chem* 1999;274:20049-52

[26] Nunez G, Benedict MA, Hu Y, Inohara N. Caspases: the proteases of the apoptotic pathway. *Oncogene* 1998;17:3237-45

[27] Miwa K, Asano M, Horai R, Iwakura Y, Nagata S, Suda T. Caspase 1-independent IL-1beta release and inflammation induced by the apoptosis inducer Fas ligand. *Nat Med* 1998;4:1287-92

[28] Hla T, Neilson K (1992) Human cyclooxygenase-2 cDNA. *Proc Natl Acad Sci* USA 89: 7384-7388

[29] Ellis EF, Chao J, Heizer ML (1989) Brain kininogen following experimental brain injury: evidence for a secondary event. *J Neurosurg* 71: 437-442

[30] Nogawa S, Zhang F, Ross ME, Iadecola C (1997) Cyclo-oxygenase-2 gene expression in neurons contributes to ischemic brain damage. *J Neurosci* 17: 2746-2755

[31] 31.Warner TD, Mitchell JA. Cyclooxygenases: new forms, new inhibitors, and lessons from the clinic. *FASEB J* 2004 5:147-157.

[32] 32.Kukar T, Murphy MP, Eriksen JL, Sagi SA, Weggen S, Smith TE, Ladd T, Khan MA, Kache R, Beard J, Dodson M, Merit S, Ozols VV, Anastasiadis PZ, Das P, Faug A, Koo EH, Golde TE. Diverse compounds mimic Alzheimer disease-causing mutatins by augmenting Abeta42 production. *Nat Med* 2005 11:545-550.

[33] Muhleisen H, Gehrmann J, Meyermann R. Reactive microglia in Creutzfeldt-Jakob disease. *Neuropathol Appl Neurobiol* 1995;21:505-17

[34] Ferrer I, Lopez E, Blanco R, Rivera R, Krupinski J, Marti E. Diffential c-Fos and caspase expression following kainic acid excitotoxicity. *Acta Neuropathol Berl* 2000;99:245-56

[35] Weller M, Rieger J, Grimmel C, VanMeir EG, DeTribolet N, Krajewski S, Reed JC, vonDeimling A, Dichgans J. Predicting chemoresistance in human malignant glioma cells: the role of molecular genetic analyses. *Int J Cancer* 1998;79:640-4

[36] Dixon EP, Stephenson DT, Clemens JA, Little SP. Bcl-Xshort is elevated following severe global ischemia in rat brains. *Brain Res* 1997;776:222-9

[37] Selznick LA, Zheng TS, Flavell RA, Rakic P, Roth KA. Amyloid beta-induced neuronal death is bax-dependent but caspase-independent. *J Neuropathol Exp Neurol* 2000;59:271-9

[38] Krajewski S, Bodrug S, Krajewska M, Shabaik A, Gascoyne R, Berean K, Reed JC. Immunohistochemical analysis of Mcl-1 protein in human tissues. Differential regulation of Mcl-1 and Bcl-2 protein production suggests a unique role for Mcl-1 in control of programmed cell death in vivo. *Am J Pathol* 1995;146:1309-19

[39] Ona VO, Li M, Vonsattel JP, Andrews LJ, Khan SQ, Chung WM, Frey AS, Menon AS, Li XJ, Stieg PE, Yuan J, Penney JB, Young AB, Cha JH, Friedlander RM. Inhibition of caspase-1 slows disease progression in a mouse model of Huntington's disease. *Nature* 1999;399:263-7

[40] Zhu SG, Sheng JG, Jones RA, Brewer MM, Zhou XQ, Mrak RE, Griffin WS. Increased interleukin-1beta converting enzyme expression and activity in Alzheimer disease. *J Neuropathol Exp Neurol* 1999;58:582-7

[41] Friedlander RM, Yuan J. ICE, neuronal apoptosis and neurodegeneration. *Cell Death Differ* 1998;5:823-31

[42] Troy CM, Rabacchi SA, Friedman WJ, Frappier TF, Brown K, Shelanski ML. Caspase-2 mediates neuronal cell death induced by beta-amyloid. *J Neurosci* 2000;20:1386-92

[43] Susin SA, Lorenzo HK, Zamzami N, Marzo I, Brenner C, Larochette N, Prevost MC, Alzari PM, Kroemer G. Mitochondrial release of caspase-2 and -9 during the apoptotic process. *J Exp Med* 1999;189:381-94

[44] Buki A, Okonkwo DO, Wang KK, Povlishock JT. Cytochrome c release and caspase activation in traumatic axonal injury. *J Neurosci* 2000;20:2825-34

[45] Hartmann A, Hunot S, Michel PP, Muriel MP, Vyas S, Faucheux BA, Mouatt-Prigent A, Turmel H, Srinivasan A, Ruberg M, Evan GI, Agid Y, Hirsch EC. Caspase-3: A vulnerability factor and final effector in apoptotic death of dopaminergic neurons in Parkinson's disease. *Proc Natl Acad Sci* USA 2000;97:2875-80

[46] Roth KA, Kuan C, Haydar TF, D'Sa-Eipper C, Shindler KS, Zheng TS, Kuida K, Flavell RA, Rakic P. Epistatic and independent functions of caspase-3 and Bcl-X(L) in developmental programmed cell death. *Proc Natl Acad Sci* USA 2000;97:466-71

[47] Krajewski S, Krajewska M, Ellerby LM, Welsh K, Xie Z, Deveraux QL, Salvesen GS, Bredesen DE, Rosenthal RE, Fiskum G, Reed JC. Release of caspase-9 from mitochondria during neuronal apoptosis and cerebral ischemia. *Proc Natl Acad Sci* USA 1999;96:5752-7

[48] LeBlanc A, Liu H, Goodyer C, Bergeron C, Hammond J. Caspase-6 role in apoptosis of human neurons, amyloidogenesis, and Alzheimer's disease. *J Biol Chem* 1999;274:23426-36

[49] Ivins KJ, Thornton PL, Rohn TT, Cotman CW. Neuronal apoptosis induced by beta-amyloid is mediated by caspase-8. *Neurobiol Dis* 1999;6:440-9

[50] Velier JJ, Ellison JA, Kikly KK, Spera PA, Barone FC, Feuerstein GZ. Caspase-8 and caspase-3 are expressed by different populations of cortical neurons undergoing delayed cell death after focal stroke in the rat. *J Neurosci* 1999;19:5932-41

[51] Fulda S, Friesen C, Los M, Scaffidi C, Mier W, Benedict M, Nunez G, Krammer PH, Peter ME, Debatin KM. Betulinic acid triggers CD95 (APO-1/Fas)- and p53-independent apoptosis via activation of caspases in neuroectodermal tumors. *Cancer Res* 1997;57:4956-64

[52] Salvesen GS. Programmed cell death and the caspases. *Apmis* 1999;107:73-79.

[53] Hengartner MO. The biochemistry of apoptosis. *Nature* 2000 407;770-776.

[54] Green DR. Apoptotic pathways: the roads to ruin. *Cell* 1998 94;695-698.

[55] Zhou H, Li Y, Liu X, Wang X. An APAF-1 cytochrome c multimeric complex is a functional apoptosome that activates procaspase-9. *J Biol Chem* 1996 86; 147-157.

[56] 56.Salgueiro-Pagadigorria CL, Kelmer-Bracht AM, Bracht A, Ishii-Iwamoto EL. Naproxen affects Ca^{2+} fluxes in mitochondria, microsomes and plasma membrane vesicles. *Chem Biol Interact* 2004;147:49-63.

[57] 57.Johnson AJ, Hsu AL, Lin HP, Song X, Chen CS. The cyclo-oxygenase-2 inhibitor celecoxib perturbs intracellular calcium by inhibiting endoplasmic reticulum Ca^{2+}-ATPases: a plausible link with its anti-tumour effect and cardiovascular risks. *Biochem J* 2002;366:831-7.

[58] Weiss H, Amberger A, Widschwendter M, Margreiter R, Ofner D, Dietl P. Inhibition of store-operated calcium entry contributes to the anti-proliferative effect of non-steroidal anti-inflammatory drugs in human colon cancer cells. *Int J Cancer* 2001;92:877–82.

[59] Berridge MJ, Bootman MD, Lipp P. Calcium—a life and death signal. *Nature* 1998;395:645–8.

[60] Pacher P, Hajnoczky G. Propagation of the apoptotic signal by mitochondrial waves. *EMBO J* 2001;20:4107–21.

[61] Li M, Wu X, Xu X-C. Induction of apoptosis in colon cancer cells by cyclooxygenase-2 inhibitor NS398 through a cytochrome *c*-dependent pathway. *Clin Cancer Res* 2001;7:1010–6.

[62] Waskewich C, Blumenthal RD, Li H, Stein R, Goldenberg DM, Burton J. Celecoxib exhibits the greatest potency amongst cyclooxygenase (COX) inhibitors for growth inhibition of COX-2-negative hematopoietic and epithelial cell lines. *Cancer Res* 2002;62:2029–33.

[63] Hsu AL, Ching TT, Wang DS, Song XQ, Rangnekar VM, Chen CS. The cyclooxygenase-2 inhibitor celecoxib induces apoptosis by blocking Akt activation in human prostate cancer cells independently of Bcl-2. *J Biol Chem* 2000;275:11397–403.

[64] Lehmann JM, Lenhard JM, Oliver BB, Ringold GM, Kliewer SA. Peroxisome proliferator-activated receptors α and γ are activated by indomethacin and other non-steroidal anti-inflammatory drugs. *J Biol Chem* 1997;272:3406–10.

[65] Yamamoto Y, Yin M-J, Lin K-M, Gaynor RB. Sulindac inhibits activation of the NF-κ B pathway. *J Biol Chem* 1999;274:27307–14.

[66] Myers C, Koki A, Pamukcu R, Wechter W, Padley RJ. Proapoptotic anti-inflammatory drugs. *Urology.* 2001 Apr;57(4 Suppl 1):73-6.

[67] Arun B, Goss P. The role of COX-2 inhibition in breast cancer treatment and prevention. *Semin Oncol.* 2004 Apr;31(2 Suppl 7):22-9.

[68] Kismet K, Akay MT, Abbasoglu O, Ercan A.Celecoxib: a potent cyclooxygenase-2 inhibitor in cancer prevention. *Cancer Detect Prev.* 2004;28(2):127-42.

[69] Sandler AB, Dubinett SM.COX-2 inhibition and lung cancer. *Semin Oncol.* 2004;31:45-52.

[70] Sinicrope FA, Gill S.Role of cyclooxygenase-2 in colorectal cancer. *Cancer Metastasis Rev.* 2004;23:63-75.

[71] Xiong HQ. Molecular targeting therapy for pancreatic cancer. *Cancer Chemother Pharmacol.* 2004;54:S69-77.

In: New Trends in Brain Research
Editor: F. J. Chen, pp. 159-173

ISBN 1-59454-834-X
© 2006 Nova Science Publishers, Inc.

Chapter VIII

REVIEW OF GENETIC MUTATIONS OF GLIOMAS IN THE MALAY POPULATION AND ITS REFLECTIONS OF TUMORIGENESIS IN SOUTH EAST ASIA

J. Abdullah[1], M. Mohd Ghazali[1], K. Asmarina[1], A. Farizan[1], N. M Isa[2] and H. Jaafar[3]

[1]Department of Neurosciences [2] Human Genome Center, [3]Department of Pathology, School of Medical Sciences, Universiti Sains Malaysia, Kubang Kerian, Kelantan, Malaysia.

ABSTRACT

Gliomas are the most common type of primary malignant brain tumors in Malaysia. Several ideas have emerged about the genetic alterations occurring in human cancers and how they contribute to tumorigenesis. The role of common genetic alterations in determining the range of individual susceptibility within the population are being increasingly recognized. The accumulation of genetic alterations are thought to drive the progression of normal cells through hyperplastic and dysplastic stages to invasive cancer and, finally, metastatic disease. With regards to that, numerous research have been aggressively carried out, focusing on the potential roles of genes which are important in cell cycle progression as well as apoptotic pathways. The results revealed *PTEN* and *p53* genes mutations to be found in mostly high grade gliomas. Loss of heterozygosity (LOH) and telomerase activities were also found in high grade glioma cases, suggesting that those actions might contribute to brain tumorigenesis in Malaysia especially amongst the Malay population. The identification of genes and pathways involved would enhance our understanding of the biology of this process. It would also provide new targets for early diagnosis and facilitate treatment design for example in developing DNA vaccine as an anti-cancer agent and virus therapy which has shown promise as a cancer treatment in Malaysia.

INTRODUCTION

Abnormal proliferation, inability of cells to die and their potential to modify their tissue environment results from accumulation of genetic aberrations [1]. The development of an invasive brain tumor involves a multistep process that has been associated with the altered expression of several oncogenes and tumor-suppressor genes. Advances in molecular biology in the past decades have revolutionized our understanding of cancer, including brain tumors. The detailed understanding of molecular events responsible for brain tumor will lead to the development of better techniques for the diagnosis and classification of human brain as well as the ultimate goal of rationally based therapy [2, 3]

A total of 21,464 cancer cases were diagnosed among Malaysians in Peninsular Malaysia in the year 2003, comprising 9,400 males and 12,064 females. A significant proportion of central nervous system neoplasms affects children in Malaysia, ranked second in incidence after leukemias with the cancer incidence per 100,000 population of 1.7 in male and 1.6 in female [4]. Gliomas are tumors of neuroepithelial origin and include the type of astrocytic tumors, oligodendroglial tumors, mixed gliomas, ependymomas and neuroepithelial tumors of uncertain origin [5]. It is the most common type of brain tumors, constituting more than 50% of all brain tumors and 2% of the malignant tumors in adults [6]. Astrocytic tumors occur in only 25% of patients in Singapore with primary brain tumors [7]. In gliomas, molecular genetic analyses play an increasing part in the classification and the treatment planning. As the largest and most important group of brain tumors, they have been receiving considerable attention from cancer geneticists.

PTEN AND LOH IN GLIOMA CASES

Among the frequently reported cases in molecular genetic research of brain tumors, *PTEN* mutations and Loss of Heterozygosity (LOH) have been suggested to play significant roles in the poor prognosis of the cancer.

In gliomas, *PTEN* gene abnormalities are preferentially found in high-grade gliomas, particularly in glioblastoma multiforme [8-12]. Deletions of the *PTEN* region at 10q23 are also reported as predominant findings in glioblastoma [11, 13, 14]. *PTEN* alterations are detectable in a low fraction (<10%) of anaplastic astrocytomas and anaplastic oligodendrogliomas and when present, indicate a poor prognosis [15].

Though association of LOH in brain tumors is not strongly correlated, frequent of allelic losses were reported in malignant astrocytoma, glioblastoma, anaplastic oligodendroglioma and ependymoma cases. In malignant astrocytoma, regular of allelic losses were defined in chromosome 10, 13q, 17p and 22q, suggesting the presence of tumor suppressor genes on this chromosomes [16]. They have also reported the LOH cases on chromosome 17p in anaplastic oligodendroglioma samples. LOH on chromosome 10 and 13q [16] were found in most anaplastic ependymoma cases. While in glioblastomas, with partial loss of chromosome 10, at least three common deletions were found which were 10q14-pter, 10q23-24 and 10q25-qter, suggestive of multiple tumor suppressor genes [17]. Forty to 60% of reported deletion in glioblastoma cases occurred on chromosome 9p21 [18].

Several studies have shown that loss of heterozygosity as well as *PTEN* mutation were correlated with poor prognosis in glioma patients [19]. They suggested that by losing function of those regions, the survival rates of the patients decreased. In our study, we found that *PTEN* mutations are infrequently reported among Malay patients. However, results showed that 21.6% of the reported *PTEN* mutations were mostly found in high grade of glioma cases [20]. Additionally, LOH was frequently occurring among Malay high grade glioma patients where 32.4% LOH was detected. Univariate Cox regression analysis revealed that histopathological grade, vascularity, *PTEN*, LOH and combined presence of *PTEN* and LOH were significant prognostic factors for the survival of patients with brain tumor in Malaysia. However, multivariate analyses indicate that no single variable was the prognostic factor for the survival [12].

TELOMERASE ACTIVITY WITH UNDETECTABLE *P16* GENE MUTATION IN GLIOMA

Another tumor suppressor gene which is frequently implicated in tumorigenesis is *p16* *(MTS1/CDKN2A/INK4A)* which is located on chromosome 9p21, which plays a major role in regulating the cell cycle at the G1–S check point. The *p16* gene was firstly demonstrated by Kamb, *et al.* in 1994. This gene composed of three exons, which encodes a 156 amino acid, 15.8-kD protein that blocks progression of cell cycle, so indirectly prevent cells from entering into the S phase through the G1 phase [22, 23]. Loss of this protein function may lead to cancer progression by allowing unregulated cellular proliferation [22].

The important role of *p16* gene in the occurrence of many types of cancer was first suggested by high frequent mutations and deletions of this gene in human cancer cell lines. Alterations of the *p16* gene are known to occur in many primary tumors through different mechanisms including homozygous deletion, point mutation, and hypermethylation of the *p16* gene promoter. PCR-SSCP (Single Strand Conformation Polymorphism) analysis was performed to screen for *p16* gene mutation at exon 1 and 2. There was no mobility shift of *p16* gene using SSCP with no mutations at exon 1 and 2 in all samples. These results suggest that another mechanism of *p16* gene alterations could be involved [20].

Recent studies have shown that activation of the telomerase is necessary for tumorigenesis. The length of the telomeres decreases due to the end replication problem with every cell division. This problem can be prevented by maintaining telomeric length. Both telomerase and telomere have been identified as targets for anticancer therapy since there were evidences of strong correlations between telomerase reactivation, cellular immortalization and cancer [24].

We detected 6 out of 23 cases (26.1%) of telomerase activities in our brain tumor samples which mostly presented as high-grade tumors. We determined telomerase activity in 23 tumor tissues base on the PCR-Telomeric Repeat Amplification Protocol (TRAP) assay using TRAP$_{EZE}$ Telomerase Detection Kit (Intergen Co., USA). Previous studies have reported similar findings of telomerase activities in glioblastoma multiforme, oligodendroglioma and medulloblastoma [25, 26]. There was a significant association between telomerase activity status and tumor grade but not with patient criteria. Telomerase activity was detected in the analyzed tumors, supporting the fact that activation of telomerase is an important feature for tumorigenesis.

P53

An important prognostic factor in gliomas is the status of the *p53* tumor-suppressor gene in the primary tumor. Alteration of the tumor suppressor gene *p53* is considered to be a critical step in the development of human cancer. It is located on chromosome 17p and has been found to influence multiple cellular functions, including progression through the cell cycle, DNA repair after radiation damage, genomic stability and also induces G1 arrest or apoptosis in a cell-type-dependent manner via the upregulation of another CDK inhibitor, *p21/WAF1.18* [27, 28].

Changes in this gene have been detected in a wide range of human tumors including gliomas and seem to be almost ubiquitous in human tumorigenesis [29]. In gliomas, the presence of *p53* gene alterations has been associated with worse prognosis. The *p53* gene often shows missense mutations in one allele and is found within exons 5 to 8 spanning the evolutionary conserved region of the protein in gliomas [30].

Forty-seven Malaysian glioma samples were analyzed using SSCP that showed *p53* mutations in 12 tumors with an incidence rate of 25.5%. Mutations were found in 2 patients of grade II, and 5 patients both in grade III and grade IV. The sequencing results revealed the presence of base-substitutions and frameshifts mutations in these glioma samples [31].

The 3 factors associated with *p53* mutations were grade, site and consistency of tumor by using univariate analysis, although multivariate analysis revealed no positive on predictors of mutation. As a conclusion although *p53* genetic alterations were involved in glioma patients in Malaysia, it has no impact on prognosis [31]. These results support the study that had been done by researchers in Singapore [7].

P27 GENE

p27 (kip1/*p27*kip1) is one of the cyclin-dependent kinase inhibitor (CDKI), which also plays important roles as a negative regulator in cell cycles [32, 33]. *p27* is encoded by CDKN1B gene, which is located on chromosome 12q13. The gene consists of three exons and is encoded for 4.99 kb of DNA.

In cell cycles, *p27* acts by binding to the cyclin-CDK complexes and inhibit their activities [34]. This disrupts the progression of G1 to S phase and leads to apoptosis of the cells [35].

Milas *et al.* (2002) reported that *p27* protein expression shows reduction after radiotherapy treatment. This was observed in several cancer cases. The same phenomenon had been identified in brain tumor cases, where a low level of *p27* protein expression during tumor progression was observed [37].

Alteration in CDKN1B gene may also contribute to dysfunction of *p27* as a tumor suppressor gene in controlling cell growth. These changes might have effect normal function and expression of the gene and increase the risk of tumor development [35] *p27* mutation was firstly reported by Morosetti *et al.* (1995). Throughout their research, they found non-sense mutation at codon 76 in adult T-lymphoma cases and homozygus deletion on exon 2 in B-immunoblastic lymphoma cases. Related to that, they suggested that *p27* mutation might have an important role in those tumor progresion. In 1996, Spirin *et al.* reported other mutations of *p27* in breast cancer. They found 2 types of mutation, a polymorphism at codon 142 and a non-sense mutation at codon 104.

Research in Malaysia found no alteration of *p27* gene in Malay glioma patients [40]. The result showed that *p27* gene alteration might have not contributed much to the development of glioma cases in Malaysia.

CYCLIN D1 GENE

Cyclin D1 encoded by *CCND1* gene and located on chromosome 11q3 [41, 42]. *CCND1* consists of 5 exons, which encodes for 259 amino acids. *CCND1* is also known as *PRAD1*, *Cyl-1, Bcl-1, U21B31, D11S287E* AND hgnc: 988 (Human Nomenclature Databases).

Cyclin D1 is classified as one of the proto-oncogen [42, 43] and is frequently associated with tumor development. Cyclin D1 protein overexpresion are frequently reported in most cancer cases including brain tumors. High level of Cyclin D1 expression will cause shortage in G1 phase and induce progression of G1 phase to S phase in cell cycles.

There are some studies done on Cyclin D1 protein overexpression and some researchers suggested that this phenomenon occurs as a result of gene amplification [44, 45]. Cyclin D1 gene amplification have frequently been suggested to contribute to the development of many cancer types including head and neck squamous cell carcinoma, cervical carcinoma and oral squamous cell carcinoma [45, 46].

Nishimoto *et al* (2004) have reported that Cyclin D1 gene polymorphism also plays important roles in the development of squamous cell carcinoma of the upper aerodigestive tract. Another study carried out by Kong *et al* (2000) found that Cyclin D1 gene polymorphism effected the age of onset of Hereditary nonpolyposis colorectal cancer.

Findings by Moreno-Bueno *et al.* (2003) proposed that mutation of *CCND1* is one of the unreported mechanisms, which also contribute to Cyclin D1 overexpression. They found that 12 bp of *CCND1* gene was deleted in endometrial cancer and they predicted this as another pathway to contribute to the development of the cancer.

Research carried out in Malaysia with the purpose of studying the role of Cyclin D1 gene in brain tumorigenesis found only one (9%) G base deletion in Malay glioma cases, suggesting that Cyclin D1 gene alteration is infrequent in the Malay population. However, the alteration of Cyclin D1 gene might play important roles in brain tumorigenesis. Base deletion of Cyclin D1 gene will lead to formation of abnormal protein which in turn, may cause cells to proliferate uncontrollably [40].

MUTATION IN PRO-APOPTOTIC GENE *BAX*

Apoptosis is an inter-related collection of pathways and mechanisms utilized to eliminate excess or unwanted cells, including neurons, in the developmental stages [50]. Pathologic roles have been defined in cancer biology. Tumor cells that inhibit apoptosis show a growth advantage over normal tissue [51]. One of the principal death-signaling pathways involves the mitochondrion, which acts by stabilizing mitochondrial function and suppressing the release of cytochrome c [52, 53]. The study of apoptosis is relevant to many aspects of cancer biology, which include tumorigenesis, tumor homeostasis, angiogenesis, metastasis and clinical treatment [54].

Bax is a strong pro-apoptotic gene that induces apoptosis, which is located on chromosome 19. It consists of six exons and a promoter region. The authors of numerous studies have attempted to address whether the mutation of *Bax* gene has a prognostic role in patients with tumors. Sequence variations in the promoter region and the coding sequence can abolish its pro-apoptotic function [55]. Mutation of *Bax* gene is also an important mechanism for loss of *Bax* expression. The *Bax* gene mutation has been suggested to play an important role in endometrial, gastric and colorectal cancers. It also has been considered as a potential tumor suppressor.[56]

In determining the potential of genetic variation in gliomas we analyzed mutation in exon 6 of *Bax* gene. Our results showed genetic alterations in 5% of our glioma sample for *Bax* gene. The alteration occurred at nucleotide 153 of *Bax* gene which resulted in C base deletion [57]. This might cause loss of Bax expression and will further enhance the escape of tumor cells from apoptotic cell death and promote malignant progression of the tumor cells.

MATRIX METALLOPROTEINASE-3 GENE VARIATION

Matrix Metalloproteinases (MMPs) are the largest group of extracellular matrix-degrading enzymes and so far 22 members have been found in human tissue [58]. MMPs are a family of closely related, metal-dependent endopeptidases. Once activated, MMPs will degrade a variety of extracellular matrix and basement membrane components [59, 60].

MMP family has substrate-specific degradation activity. Specifically, Matrix Metalloproteinse-3 (MMP-3) acts on type IV collagen that forms basal membrane [61]. Expression of most MMPs is normally low in tissues and is induced when remodelling of extracellular matrix is required. Numerous studies have shown that a high expression of MMPs in brain tumors is correlated with an increased aggressiveness of tumors.

Recently, a naturally occurring sequence variation in the human *MMP-3* gene promoter has been reported [62]. *MMP-3* gene maps on chromosome 11, at 11q22.3. MMP-3 gene encoded matrix metalloproteinase-3 which also known as stromelysin 1 or progelatinase. Changes in MMP-3 biosynthesis usually proceed with changes in gene transcription and at the mRNA level. The insertion of an A in the MMP-3 gene promoter sequence halves its transcription activity.

It has been described that there are functional polymorphism at position -1171 bp upstream from the start of the transcription of promoter sequence MMP-3 gene, consisting in a stretch of five or six adenosines [63]. In vitro assays of promoter activity showed that 5A allele had 2-fold higher promoter activity than the 6A allele. The polymorphism that has been recently tested would enhance cancers susceptibility in lymphatic metastasis of non-small cell lung carcinoma, renal cell carcinoma, breast, ovarian and colorectal cancer [62, 64-66]. It was, however, unclear whether the 5A/6A polymorphism plays a role in the regulation of stromelysin-1 expression in gliomas. Our study showed those 5A alleles were detected in more than 80% of our glioma samples [67].

RAS, C-MYC AND EGFR

Ras gene families consists of 3 members: N-ras, H-ras and K-ras, which encodes for the highly homologous protein so called p21 according to their molecular weight. The inactivation of ras gene by point mutation are the most frequent and it is well known that in genetics an alteration can be associated with human cancers including brain tumors. Common mechanisms of inactivation of these genes are missense mutations at the well known hot spot codon 12, 13 and 16 [68]. Activating point mutations have been localized in codons 12, 13, 59, 61, 63, 116,117, 119 and 146 [69]. All these alterations occur at or near the guanine nucleotide biding sites.

The presence of *ras* mutation has also been shown to be significant in terms of prognosis. Considering it's importance, the ras gene might be the good target for the development of anticancer therapy [70]. Our results revealed that no ras mutations were present when using PCR-SSCP analyses in the DNA extracted from our gliomas tissues.

According to Yusoff et al (2004), Zan et al (2003) and Ghazali et al (2005), there were no *ras* mutations detected in all tumour analyzed from Malaysian patients [71-73]. They concluded that these genes did not play a major role in tumourgenesis mainly in malignant gliomas. A previous study which involved direct sequencing analysis in oral tumours also reported that no mutation were found in *N-ras, K-ras* and *H-ras* genes [74]. Activating *ras* mutations can be found in human malignancies with an overall frequency of 15-20%. A high incidence of *ras* gene mutations has been reported in malignant tumors of the pancreas (80-90%, K-ras), in colorectal carcinomas (30-60%), in non-melanoma skin cancer (30-50%, H-ras), in hematopoietic neoplasia of myeloid origin (18-30%, K-and N-ras) and in seminoma (25-40%, K-ras) [75]. In other tumors, a mutant *ras* gene is found at a lower frequency: in breast carcinoma (0-12%, K-ras), glioblastoma and neuroblastoma (0-10%, K-and N-ras) [69].

The *c-myc* gene was discovered as the cellular homolog of the retroviral v-myc oncogene 20 years ago [76, 77]. The c-myc proto-oncogene was subsequently found to be activated in various animal and human tumors [78-80]. It belonged to the family of *myc* gene that included B-myc, L-myc, N-myc and s-myc; however only c-myc, L-myc and N-myc have had neoplastic potential [81].

The *c-myc* gene, mapped on human chromosome 8q24, encodes the transcription factor c-Myc, which heterodimerizes with a partner protein, Max, to regulate gene expression. The amplification of the n-myc gene in neuroblastomas appears to correlate with the clinical stage of the tumor and with the poor prognosis of the patients. Therefore it is tempting to speculate that the n-myc protein is one of the essential products necessary for the aberrant behavior of neuroblastoma cells [82].

c-Myc's status as an important target was reinforced by a recent widely-reported paper published in Science by Dean Felsher at Stanford, in which he demonstrated that a temporary reduction in c-Myc expression followed by reactivation, in a genetically engineered mouse model, induced highly selective and complete apoptosis in cancer cells, while having no effect on normal cells [83].

In human cancers, the *c-myc* gene is activated through several mechanisms. Investigation of *c-myc* gene alterations in glioma may provide important knowledge about the genetic basis which is based on fact that alteration in *c-myc* gene may contribute to the overexpression and amplification of c-Myc [84]. The frequency of genetic alterations of c-myc in human cancer [80] has allowed estimation that approximately 70,000 US cancer deaths per year are associated with changes in the c-myc gene or its expression. C-myc may contribute to one-seventh of US cancer deaths, recent efforts have been directed towards understanding the function of the c-myc protein in cancer biology with the hope that therapeutic insights will emerge [76, 85, 86]. The *c-myc* gene is amplified in various human cancers such as lung carcinoma [87], breast carcinoma [88] and rare cases of colon carcinoma [89]. Ghazali et al (2005) showed that no abnormal migration shifts were detected in the entire glioma sample analyzed for mutation on c-myc in North East Malaysian patients using the PCR-SSCP technique [86].

Molecular abnormalities associated with primary brain tumors include a wide variety of changes in tumor suppressor gene, proto-oncogenes and growth factors. The *EGFR* gene is a multifocal allosteric transmembrane protein with an intra cellular binding site for EGF, and acts as a tyrosine kinase. The gene is localized on the short arm of chromosome 7, within 7p11 – 13, and is called erb – B1. This receptor has been found to be over-expressed in 50% to 70% of glioblastoma multiforme. Although the functions of the proteins encoded by the most proto-oncogenes are not precisely known, biochemical activities of several proto-oncogene products have been identified. Some of the gene products are identical or related to, proteins, known to be important in growth regulation.

The current interests of molecular abnormalities in brain tumours have led our group to study *EGFR* gene mutation in relation to gliomas occurrence. In determining the genetic variations in *EGFR* genes, glioma samples were subjected to polymerase chain reaction (PCR). Amplified products were then directly sequenced. The results revealed no *EGFR* gene alterations were found in all of our glioma samples.

According to a the previous study, *EGFR* gene was often mutated in high-grade gliomas in adults, but the frequency of EGFR mutations was still low. Ghazali et al (2005) indicated that there was no alteration of *EGFR* gene via PCR-SSCP and point mutation in exon 1 from Malaysian patients and this gene might not play a major role in tumourigenesis [86]. David et al found that *EGFR* gene amplifications does not occur in Pleomorphic xanthoastrocytoma (PXA) but glioblastoma multiformee (GBM) that arise from PXA may display *EGFR* gene amplification. In adult gangliogliomas, another benign form of astrocytic glioma, *EGFR* gene amplification or allelic loss on chromosomes 10, 13q, 17p, 19q and 22q was not detected.

In simple logistic regression analysis of all three genes analyzed where there were no alteration of ras, c-myc and EGFR, clinical and radiological variables which were found to be significant were hemiplegia (Crude OR 23.29, 95% CI 2.84- 225.45, p=0.004), vascularity (Crude OR = 5.5, 95% CI 1.03 – 29.48, p=0.047) and response to radiotherapy (Crude OR=13.75, 95% CI 2.47-76.42, p=0.003). For those who were hemiplegic, they were 25 times more likely to have a high pathological grade compared to those without hemiplegia. Patients with vascular involvement were 5.5 times more likely to have higher pathological grade. However, this finding was not significant in multivariate analysis. Patients who had radiotherapy were nearly 14 times more likely to have higher pathological grade.

Multivariate analysis revealed that patients with hemiplegia were more likely to have higher pathological grade (adjusted OR =171.36, 95% CI 388 – 7566.01, p= 0.008). For those who had higher pathological grading were 80 times more likely to have radiotherapy (adjusted OR 80.92, 95% CI 3.94-1662.91, p=0.004). Other variables were found as insignificant. Our Malaysian patients with malignant gliomas, studied with no ras, c-myc and EGFR mutations, are still alive 6 years after treatment.

CONCLUSION AND FUTURE DIRECTIONS

Multiple genetic alterations are sequentially occurring in carcinogenesis of many cancer types including brain tumors. Many of the abnormalities usually lead to the loss of normal progress through cell cycle and overexpression of growth factors and/or their receptors. In addition, a number of genetic abnormalities have been listed, where the alterations of the markers are hopefully bringing new information on value of prognostication towards the patient's response to treatment.

Based on a cancer survey in Malaysia, brain tumors are the second most frequently reported cases, after leukaemia in children. The adult brain tumor cases are reported to have a crude increment of about 2000 new cases every year [90]. With regards to that, current research and findings are hopefully helpful in developing new approaches to treat brain tumors in Malaysian and South East Asian patients.

In recent years, gene therapy has become one of the most evolving therapeutic modality for malignant gliomas. With the neural stem cell-guided gene therapy, this approach could be significantly enhanced. *PTEN*, LOH and p53 could be among the targeted genes for therapy in malignant gliomas since those genes have showed frequent alterations among Malay patients and hopefully other South East Asian patients since the population is homogenously from the same anthropological stock. Besides that, a high frequency of telomerase activities in high grade gliomas patients were detected suggesting their importance in brain tumorigenesis. Antisense therapy for telomerase is one of the promising treatments which have been developed by a group of researchers [91] to inhibit human telomeric activities. Other malignant gliomas therapies which are being developed including oncolytic virus therapies [92, 93], angiogenesis inhibitor and neural stem cells. These are among the future promising approaches that could be universally applied.

Further investigations should be done to determine other brain tumor markers which could be useful for therapeutic purposes. This review opefully provides important knowledge of central nervous system tumour etiologies which are important for the development of prevention strategies. It is hope that more data will come out from South East Asian countries in the near future via a close and cohort collaboration.

ACKNOWLEDGEMENT

We would like to acknowledge Majlis Kanser Nasional (MAKNA) for the grants supporting the studies of *c-Myc, Ras, EGFR, NF2, Bax, MMP-3, p27* and *Cyclin D1* genes, the short term grant under the Intensification of Research in Priority Areas (IRPA) for *PTEN* and LOH studies (No. 304/PPSP/6131122), FELDA Foundation for the support of *p16* and telomerase studies (No. 304/PPSP/6150033Y104), and The Malaysian Toray Research Foundation Grant for *p53* gene study (No. 380/0500/5051). We would also like to acknowledge Professor Mohd Nizam Isa who was directly involved in these IRPA projects until the year 2002.

REFERENCES

[1]   Santarius T, Kirsch M, Rossi ML, Black PM. Molecular aspects of neuro-oncology. *Clin Neurol Neurosurg* 1997;99(3):184-95.

[2]   Michael D. Taylor KTJTR. Neurogenetics and the molecular biology of human brain tumors. In: JR AHKERL, editor. *Brain Tumors An encyclopaedic approach*. London: Churchill Livingstone; 2001. p. 71-103.

[3]   Hilton DA, Melling C. Genetic markers in the assessment of intrinsic brain tumours. *Current Diagnostic Pathology* 2004;10: 83–92.

[4]   Lim G, Halimah Y, editors. Second Report of the National Cancer Registry. Cancer Incidence in Malaysia 2003. 2 ed: *National Cancer Registry*. Kuala Lumpur; 2004.

[5]   Kleihues P, Louis DN, Scheithauer BW, Rorke LB, Reifenberger G, Burger PC, et al. The WHO classification of tumors of the nervous system. *J Neuropathol Exp Neurol* 2002;61(3):215-25; discussion 226-9.

[6]   Phatak P, Selvi SK, Divya T, Hegde AS, Hegde S, Somasundaram K. Alterations in tumour suppressor gene p53 in human gliomas from Indian patients. *J Biosci* 2002;27(7):673-8.

[7]   Das A, Tan WL, Teo J, Smith DR. Glioblastoma multiformee in an Asian population: evidence for a distinct genetic pathway. *J Neurooncol* 2002;60(2):117-25.

[8]   Davies MP, Gibbs FE, Halliwell N, Joyce KA, Roebuck MM, Rossi ML, et al. Mutation in the *PTEN*/MMAC1 gene in archival low grade and high grade gliomas. *Br J Cancer* 1999;79(9-10):1542-8.

[9]   Hill JR, Kuriyama N, Kuriyama H, Israel MA. Molecular genetics of brain tumors. *Arch Neurol* 1999;56(4):439-41.

[10]   Maier D, Zhang Z, Taylor E, Hamou MF, Gratzl O, Van Meir EG, et al. Somatic deletion mapping on chromosome 10 and sequence analysis of *PTEN*/MMAC1 point to the 10q25-26 region as the primary target in low-grade and high-grade gliomas. *Oncogene* 1998;16(25):3331-5.

[11]   Rasheed BK, Stenzel TT, McLendon RE, Parsons R, Friedman AH, Friedman HS, et al. *PTEN* gene mutations are seen in high-grade but not in low-grade gliomas. *Cancer Res* 1997;57(19):4187-90.

[12]   Zainuddin N, Jaafar H, Isa MN, Abdullah JM. Presence of allelic loss and *PTEN* mutations in malignant gliomas from Malay patients. *Med J Malaysia* 2004;59(4):468-79.

[13]   Li J, Yen C, Liaw D, Podsypanina K, Bose S, Wang SI, et al. *PTEN*, a putative protein tyrosine phosphatase gene mutated in human brain, breast, and prostate cancer. *Science* 1997;275(5308):1943-7.

[14] Wang SI, Puc J, Li J, Bruce JN, Cairns P, Sidransky D, et al. Somatic mutations of *PTEN* in glioblastoma multiformee. *Cancer Res* 1997;57(19):4183-6.

[15] Knobbe CB, Merlo A, Reifenberger G. Pten signaling in gliomas. *Neuro-oncol* 2002;4(3):196-211.

[16] Lee SH, Kim JH, Rhee CH, Kang YS, Lee JH, Hong SI, et al. Loss of heterozygosity on chromosome 10, 13q(Rb), 17p, and p53 gene mutations in human brain gliomas. *J Korean Med Sci* 1995;10(6):442-8.

[17] Fujisawa H, Reis RM, Nakamura M, Colella S, Yonekawa Y, Kleihues P, et al. Loss of heterozygosity on chromosome 10 is more extensive in primary (de novo) than in secondary glioblastomas. *Lab Invest* 2000;80(1):65-72.

[18] Cheng Y, Ng HK, Ding M, Zhang SF, Pang JC, Lo KW. Molecular analysis of microdissected de novo glioblastomas and paired astrocytic tumors. *J Neuropathol Exp Neurol* 1999;58(2):120-8.

[19] Balesaria S, Brock C, Bower M, Clark J, Nicholson SK, Lewis P, et al. Loss of chromosome 10 is an independent prognostic factor in high-grade gliomas. *Br J Cancer* 1999;81(8):1371-7.

[20] Abdullah JM, Zainuddin N, Sulong S, Jaafar H, Isa MN. Molecular genetic analysis of phosphatase and tensin homolog and p16 tumor suppressor genes in patients with malignant glioma. *Neurosurg Focus* 2003;14(4):e6.

[21] Kamb A, Gruis NA, Weaver-Feldhaus J, Liu Q, Harshman K, Tavtigian SV, et al. A cell cycle regulator potentially involved in genesis of many tumor types. *Science* 1994;264(5157):436-40.

[22] Liggett WH, Jr., Sidransky D. Role of the p16 tumor suppressor gene in cancer. *J Clin Oncol* 1998;16(3):1197-206.

[23] Guang Z, Xianhou Y. Study of deletion of P16 gene in the progression of brain astrocytomas. *Chinese J Cancer Res* 1998;10:412-417.

[24] Urquidi V, Tarin D, Goodison S. Role of telomerase in cell senescence and oncogenesis. *Annu Rev Med* 2000;51:65-79.

[25] Chen HJ, Cho CL, Liang CL, Chen L, Chang HW, Lu K, et al. Differential telomerase expression and telomere length in primary intracranial tumors. *Chang Gung Med J* 2001;24(6):352-60.

[26] Sano T, Asai A, Mishima K, Fujimaki T, Kirino T. Telomerase activity in 144 brain tumours. *Br J Cancer* 1998;77(10):1633-7.

[27] Lane DP. Cancer. p53, guardian of the genome. *Nature* 1992;358(6381):15-6.

[28] Hussain SA, James ND. Molecular markers in bladder cancer. *Semin Radiat Oncol* 2005;15(1):3-9.

[29] Patt S, Gries H, Giraldo M, Cervos-Navarro J, Martin H, Janisch W, et al. p53 gene mutations in human astrocytic brain tumors including pilocytic astrocytomas. *Hum Pathol* 1996;27(6):586-9.

[30] Greenblatt MS, Bennett WP, Hollstein M, Harris CC. Mutations in the p53 tumor suppressor gene: clues to cancer etiology and molecular pathogenesis. *Cancer Res* 1994;54(18):4855-78.

[31] Yusoff AA, Abdullah J, Abdullah MR, Mohd Ariff AR, Isa MN. Association of p53 tumor suppressor gene with paraclinical and clinical modalities of gliomas patients in Malaysia. *Acta Neurochir* (Wien) 2004;146(6):595-601.

[32]   Ferrando AA, Balbin M, Pendas AM, Vizoso F, Velasco G, Lopez-Otin C. Mutational analysis of the human cyclin-dependent kinase inhibitor *p27*kip1 in primary breast carcinomas. *Hum Genet* 1996;97(1):91-4.

[33]   Shin JY, Kim HS, Lee KS, Kim J, Park JB, Won MH, et al. Mutation and expression of the *p27*KIP1 and p57KIP2 genes in human gastric cancer. *Exp Mol Med* 2000;32(2):79-83.

[34]   Coqueret O. New roles for p21 and *p27* cell-cycle inhibitors: a function for each cell compartment? *Trends Cell Biol* 2003;13(2):65-70.

[35]   Kang YK, Kim WH, Jang JJ. Expression of G1-S modulators (p53, p16, *p27*, cyclin D1, Rb) and Smad4/Dpc4 in intrahepatic cholangiocarcinoma. *Hum Pathol* 2002;33(9):877-83.

[36]   Milas L, Akimoto T, Hunter NR, Mason KA, Buchmiller L, Yamakawa M, et al. Relationship between cyclin D1 expression and poor radioresponse of murine carcinomas. *Int J Radiat Oncol Biol Phys* 2002;52(2):514-21.

[37]   Piva R, Cavalla P, Bortolotto S, Cordera S, Richiardi P, Schiffer D. *p27*/kip1 expression in human astrocytic gliomas. *Neurosci Lett* 1997;234(2-3):127-30.

[38]   Morosetti R, Kawamata N, Gombart AF, Miller CW, Hatta Y, Hirama T, et al. Alterations of the *p27*KIP1 gene in non-Hodgkin's lymphomas and adult T-cell leukemia/lymphoma. *Blood* 1995;86(5):1924-30.

[39]   Spirin KS, Simpson JF, Takeuchi S, Kawamata N, Miller CW, Koeffler HP. *p27*/Kip1 mutation found in breast cancer. *Cancer Res* 1996;56(10):2400-4.

[40]   Farizan A, Asmarina K, Abdullah J, Jaafar H, Ghazali MM, Aini I, et al. Screening of Cyclin Dependent Kinase Inhibitor *p27* and Cyclin D1 gene in association with gliomas and meningiomas in Malaysia. *The Malaysian Journal of Medical Sciences* 2005;12:240.

[41]   Shigemasa K, Tanimoto H, Parham GP, Parmley TH, Ohama K, O'Brien TJ. Cyclin D1 overexpression and p53 mutation status in epithelial ovarian cancer. *J Soc Gynecol Investig* 1999;6(2):102-8.

[42]   Sundarrajan M, Gupta S, Rao KV. Overexpression of cyclin D1 is associated with the decondensation of chromatin during den-induced sequential hepatocarcinogenesis. *Cell Biol Int* 2002;26(8):699-706.

[43]   Cordon-Cardo C. Mutations of cell cycle regulators. Biological and clinical implications for human neoplasia. *Am J Pathol* 1995;147(3):545-60.

[44]   Koontongkaew S, Chareonkitkajorn L, Chanvitan A, Leelakriangsak M, Amornphimoltham P. Alterations of p53, pRb, cyclin D(1) and cdk4 in human oral and pharyngeal squamous cell carcinomas. *Oral Oncol* 2000;36(4):334-9.

[45]   Rousseau A, Lim MS, Lin Z, Jordan RC. Frequent cyclin D1 gene amplification and protein overexpression in oral epithelial dysplasias. *Oral Oncol* 2001;37(3):268-75.

[46]   Cheung TH, Yu MM, Lo KW, Yim SF, Chung TK, Wong YF. Alteration of cyclin D1 and CDK4 gene in carcinoma of uterine cervix. *Cancer Lett* 2001;166(2):199-206.

[47]   Nishimoto IN, Pinheiro NA, Rogatto SR, Carvalho AL, Simpson AJ, Caballero OL, et al. Cyclin D1 gene polymorphism as a risk factor for squamous cell carcinoma of the upper aerodigestive system in non-alcoholics. *Oral Oncol* 2004;40(6):604-10.

[48]   Kong S, Amos CI, Luthra R, Lynch PM, Levin B, Frazier ML. Effects of cyclin D1 polymorphism on age of onset of hereditary nonpolyposis colorectal cancer. *Cancer Res* 2000;60(2):249-52.

[49] Moreno-Bueno G, Rodriguez-Perales S, Sanchez-Estevez C, Hardisson D, Sarrio D, Prat J, et al. Cyclin D1 gene (CCND1) mutations in endometrial cancer. *Oncogene* 2003;22(38):6115-8.

[50] Liou AK, Clark RS, Henshall DC, Yin XM, Chen J. To die or not to die for neurons in ischemia, traumatic brain injury and epilepsy: a review on the stress-activated signaling pathways and apoptotic pathways. *Prog Neurobiol* 2003;69(2):103-42.

[51] Bast BT, Pogrel MA, Regezi JA. The expression of apoptotic proteins and matrix metalloproteinases in odontogenic myxomas. *J Oral Maxillofac Surg* 2003;61(12):1463-6.

[52] Evan GI, Vousden KH. Proliferation, cell cycle and apoptosis in cancer. *Nature* 2001;411(6835):342-8.

[53] Kuhlmann T, Glas M, zum Bruch C, Mueller W, Weber A, Zipp F, et al. Investigation of bax, bcl-2, bcl-x and p53 gene polymorphisms in multiple sclerosis. *J Neuroimmunol* 2002;129(1-2):154-60.

[54] McGill G, Fisher DE. Apoptosis in tumorigenesis and cancer therapy. *Front Biosci* 1997;2:d353-79.

[55] Rampino N, Yamamoto H, Ionov Y, Li Y, Sawai H, Reed JC, et al. Somatic frameshift mutations in the BAX gene in colon cancers of the microsatellite mutator phenotype. *Science* 1997;275(5302):967-9.

[56] Sakuragi N, Salah-eldin AE, Watari H, Itoh T, Inoue S, Moriuchi T, et al. Bax, Bcl-2, and p53 expression in endometrial cancer. *Gynecol Oncol* 2002;86(3):288-96.

[57] Asmarina K, Abdullah J, Jaafar H, Aini I, Manaf A. Alteration of Bax gene in brain tumors. *Journal of Clinical Neuroscience* 2004;11(supplement 1):S103.

[58] Levicar N, Nuttall RK, Lah TT. Proteases in brain tumour progression. *Acta Neurochir* (Wien) 2003;145(9):825-38.

[59] McCawley LJ, Matrisian LM. Matrix metalloproteinases: multifunctional contributors to tumor progression. *Mol Med Today* 2000;6(4):149-56.

[60] Curran S, Murray GI. Matrix metalloproteinases: molecular aspects of their roles in tumour invasion and metastasis. *Eur J Cancer* 2000;36(13 Spec No):1621-30.

[61] Ghilardi G, Biondi ML, Mangoni J, Leviti S, DeMonti M, Guagnellini E, et al. Matrix metalloproteinase-1 promoter polymorphism 1G/2G is correlated with colorectal cancer invasiveness. *Clin Cancer Res* 2001;7(8):2344-6.

[62] Fang S, Jin X, Wang R, Li Y, Guo W, Wang N, et al. Polymorphisms in the MMP1 and MMP3 promoter and non-small cell lung carcinoma in North China. *Carcinogenesis* 2005;26(2):481-6.

[63] Ye S, Eriksson P, Hamsten A, Kurkinen M, Humphries SE, Henney AM. Progression of coronary atherosclerosis is associated with a common genetic variant of the human stromelysin-1 promoter which results in reduced gene expression. *J Biol Chem* 1996;271(22):13055-60.

[64] Ghilardi G, Biondi ML, Caputo M, Leviti S, DeMonti M, Guagnellini E, et al. A single nucleotide polymorphism in the matrix metalloproteinase-3 promoter enhances breast cancer susceptibility. *Clin Cancer Res* 2002;8(12):3820-3.

[65] Hirata H, Okayama N, Naito K, Inoue R, Yoshihiro S, Matsuyama H, et al. Association of a haplotype of matrix metalloproteinase (MMP)-1 and MMP-3 polymorphisms with renal cell carcinoma. *Carcinogenesis* 2004;25(12):2379-84.

[66] Smolarz B, Szyllo K, Romanowicz-Makowska H, Niewiadomski M, Kozlowska E, Kulig A. PCR analysis of matrix metalloproteinase 3 (MMP-3) gene promoter polymorphism in ovarian cancer. *Pol J Pathol* 2003;54(4):233-8.

[67] Asmarina K, Abdullah J, Farizan A, Jaafar H, Ghazali MM, Aini I, et al. Preliminary Report Of Genetic Variation In Human Stromelysin 1 Promoter In Gliomas And Meningiomas. In: 6th National Congress on Genetics; 2005; *Kuala Lumpur* (Malaysia); 2005. p. 192-193.

[68] Gomori E, Doczi T, Pajor L, Matolcsy A. Sporadic p53 mutations and absence of ras mutations in glioblastomas. *Acta Neurochir* (Wien) 1999;141(6):593-9.

[69] Watzinger F, Lion T. RAS family. *In: Atlas of genetics and cytogenetics in oncology and haematology*; 1999.

[70] Isobe T, Hiyama K, Yoshida Y, Fujiwara Y, Yamakido M. Prognostic significance of p53 and ras gene abnormalities in lung adenocarcinoma patients with stage I disease after curative resection. *Jpn J Cancer Res* 1994;85(12):1240-6.

[71] Yusoff AA, J.Abdullah, H.Jaafar, Aini I, Manaf A, Khatijah Y, et al. The lack of a role for ras gene in human gliomas in Malaysian patients. *The Malaysian Journal of Medical Sciences*, 2004;11(1):145.

[72] Zan MSM, Fauzi ARM, Yusoff AA, Ghazali MM, Abdullah J, Aini I, et al. Molecular Studies of NF2 and Ras Family Gene in Malaysian Human Brain Tumors. *Med J Malaysia* 2003.;58 (Supplement E):102.

[73] Ghazali MM, Zan MSM, Fauzi ARM, Yusoff AA, Abdullah J, Aini I, et al. Ras, c-myc and epidermal growth factor receptor (EGFR) gene alteration in human gliomas in North East Malaysian patients. *The Malaysian Journal of Medical Sciences*, 2005;12(Suppl 1):161.

[74] SÜZEN S, PARRY JM. Analysis of ras Gene Mutation in Human Oral Tumours by Polymerase Chain Reaction and Direct Sequencing. *Tr. J. of Med. Sci.* 2001;31:217-223.

[75] Halter SA, Webb L, Rose J. Lack of ras mutations and prediction of long-term survival in carcinoma of the colon. *Mod Pathol* 1992;5(2):131-4.

[76] Bishop JM. Retroviruses and cancer genes. *Adv.Cancer Res* 1982;37:1-32.

[77] Sheiness D, L.Fanshier, Bishop JM. Identification of nucleotide sequences which may encode the oncogenic capacity of avian retrovirus MC29. *J.Virol* 1978;28:600-610.

[78] Cole MD. The myc oncogene; its role in transformation and differentiation. *Annu.Rev.Genet.* 1986;20:361-384.

[79] Dalla-Favera, R EPG, S.Martinotti, G.Faranchini, T.S.Papas, Gallo RC, et al. Cloning and characterization of different human sequences related to the onc gene (v-myc) of avian myelocytomatosis virus (MC29). *Proc. Natl. Acad. Sci* USA 1982;79: 6497-6501.

[80] Dang CV, L.A.Lee. *c-myc function in neoplasia*. R.G. Landes and Springer-Verlag, Austin, Tex. 1995.

[81] Facchini LM, Penn LZ. The molecular role of Myc in growth and transformation: recent discoveries lead to new insights. *Faseb J* 1998;12(9):633-51.

[82] Peng H, Diss T, Isaacson PG, Pan L. c-myc gene abnormalities in mucosa-associated lymphoid tissue (MALT) lymphomas. *J Pathol* 1997;181(4):381-6.

[83] Jain M, Arvanitis C, Chu K, Dewey W, Leonhardt E, Trinh M, et al. Sustained loss of a neoplastic phenotype by brief inactivation of MYC. *Science* 2002;297(5578):102-4.

[84] Peng H, Du M, Ji J, Isaacson PG, Pan L. High-resolution SSCP analysis using polyacrylamide agarose composite gel and a background-free silver staining method. *Biotechniques* 1995;19(3):410-4.

[85] Blackwood EM, R.N.Eisenman. Myc and Max function as a nucleoprotein complex. *Curr. Opin. Genet. Dev.* 1991; 2:227-235.

[86] Mazira Mohamad Ghazali, Shahril Mohd Zan, Abdul Aziz Yusoff, Jafri Abdullah, Hasnan Jaafar, Abdul Rahman Arif et al. Absence of ras, c-myc and Epidermal Growth Factor Receptor (EGFR) mutation in human gliomas in the North East Malaysian patients and its clinical factors associated with pathological grading after 5 years of diagnosis. *Malaysian Journal of Medical Sciences.* 2005; 12 (2): 27-33

[87] Little CD, Nau MM, Carney DN, Gazdar AF, J.D.Minna. Amplification and expression of the c-myc oncogene in human lung cancer cell lines. *Nature* 1983; 306:194-196.

[88] Munzel P, D.Marx, H.Kochel, A.Schauer, K.W.Bock. Genomic alterations of the c-myc protooncogene in relation to the overexpression of c-erbB2 and Ki-67 in human breast and cervix carcinomas. *J Cancer Res. Clin. Oncol* 1991;117: 603-607.

[89] Augenlicht LH, S.Wadler, G.Corner, C.Richards, L.Ryan, A.S.Multani, et al. Low-level c-myc amplification in human colonic carcinoma cell lines and tumors: a frequent, p53-independent mutation associated with improved outcome in a randomized multi-institutional trial. *Cancer Res.* 1997; 57:1769-1775.

[90] Malaysia Ministry of Health. *Annual report.* 1999.

[91] Kanzawa T, Ito H, Kondo Y, Kondo S. Current and Future Gene Therapy for Malignant Gliomas. *J Biomed Biotechnol* 2003; 1:25-34.

[92] Abdul Rahman Omar, Aini Ideris, Abdul Manaf Ali, Fauziah Othman, Khatijah Yusoff, Jafri Malin Abdullah, Haryati Shila Mohamad Wali, Madihah Zawawi and Narayani Meyyappan. An overview on the development of Newcastle disease virus as an anti-cancer therapy. *Malaysian Journal of Medical Sciences.* 2003; 10: 4-12

[93] Mohd Azmi Mohd Lila, John Shia Kwong Siew, Hayati Zakaria, Suria Mohd Saad, Lim Shen Ni and Jafri Malin Abdullah. Cell Targeting in Anti-Cancer Gene Therapy. *Malaysian Journal of Medical Sciences.* 2004; 11: 9-23

In: New Trends in Brain Research
Editor: F. J. Chen, pp. 175-199

ISBN 1-59454-834-X
© 2006 Nova Science Publishers, Inc.

Chapter IX

REGISTRATION OF OPTICAL TOPOGRAPHIC MAPS AND MAGNETIC RESONANCE IMAGING

Michel Mourad[1], Malek Adjouadi[1], Melvin Ayala[1] and Ilker Yaylali[2]
[1]Department of Electrical & Computer Engineering,
Florida International University, Miami, Florida
[2]Department of Neurology, Miami Children's Hospital, Miami, Florida

ABSTRACT

This paper presents a methodology for functional brain mapping through the integration of optical topographic maps (OTM) with anatomical magnetic resonance imaging (MRI). The topographic images are mapped to both the skull and cortical surface of the brain. Eight subjects underwent an MRI and optical topography system (OTS) exams, during which anatomical MR images and optical topographic maps were acquired. In order to map the motor functional areas in the brain, a functional experiment is performed by using the ETG-100 OTS and is based on a repeated finger-tapping task alternated with relaxed states. The integration process involves estimating the probes location on the MRI head model and warping the 2D topographic images on the 3D MRI head/brain model. After integrating OTS with MRI a movie depicting the changes of the brain activation is played on the MRI head model. A graphical user interface (GUI) is developed to integrate the above modalities and serve as an application platform for neuroscience studies and for assisting neurosurgeons at localizing key functional regions in the brain.

Keywords: Optical Topographic Maps, Magnetic resonance imaging (MRI), Source Localization, and Image Registration.

1Florida International University, 10555 W. Flagler Street, Miami FL 33174Tel: (305) 348-3019, mourad.mourad@fiu.edu, adjouadi@fiu.edu, melvin.ayala@fiu.edu

2Miami Children's Hospital, 3100 S.W. 62nd Avenue, Miami, Fl 33155, Tel: (305) 663-8504 Emails: Ilker.Yaylali@mch.com

1. INTRODUCTION

The diagnostic brain imaging can be classified into two major domains: (1) structural imaging assess volume structure of the brain to analyze its anatomy; and (2) functional imaging assess brain function using biochemical, electrical, or physiological properties of the brain in order to map, measure and localize brain activity. Structural imaging thus provides information about the anatomy of the brain. On the other hand, the goal of functional imaging is to provide information on the physiological state of the cerebral tissue.

In recent years, there have been significant efforts to develop algorithms for optical image reconstruction with the objectives to enhance image sensitivity and resolution [Arridge 1999; Boas et al. 2004]. Recent articles [Zhang et al. 2005; Boas et al. 2005; Strangman et al. 2002; Kleinschmidt et al 1996] have also investigated the merits of integrating diffuse optical tomography or NIRS and magnetic resonance imaging of the human brain.

Functional imaging modalities such as the ones used in this study (MRI and OTS) have a wide range of clinical applications. Because it provides convenient brain function measurements, OTS can be used for measuring various brain functions, such as motor and sensory functions, visual and auditory functions, and high order functions related to language and consciousness, and for the measurement of the visual cortex during sleep [Kennan et al, 2002; Frostig et al, 1990; Mayhew et al, 1998].

The proposed research has been conducted by using OTS and MRI machines in synergy. The main objective of the study was to superimpose the topographic image generated by OTS on the 3D MRI head model and be able to validate the results by using a simple test of finger tapping. This integrated process is designed to enable researchers and clinicians to localize on the structural MRI the activation seen through the topographic image.

The integrated OTS-MRI process consisted of the following steps:

- Collect brain functional data on both MRI and OTS modalities from eight subjects during a finger tapping task.The same test was administered to each subject.
- Create the topographic image from the samples of data generated by the OTS.
- Threshold the MRI slices using basic global thresholding algorithm
- Generate 3D head models from the structural MRI after smooth rendering the thresholded MRI slices. Note that the basic global thresholding algorithm is used to effectively threshold the MRI slices prior to the 3D rendering.
- Identify the region on the 3D MRI head model from which the topographic image generated by OTS was taken.
- Register the topographic image to the 3D head model.
- Extract brain structure from MRI slices
- Project the resulting warped topographic maps from the skull onto the cortical surface.

2. OPTICAL TOPOGRAPHY SYSTEM

2.1 Measurement Principle

The OTS sends a near infrared light of about 1.5mW from optical fibers attached to the scalp. Then the light penetrates the skull reaching the cerebral cortex. It can penetrate to a depth of about 3 cm, and then scatter by hemoglobin in the blood. Some of the light is partially reflected back to the scalp and is detected at a distance of 3cm from the source across the scalp, the detected light passes through the regions inside the skull as illustrated in Figure 1. Then it is sent through optical fibers and detected with a sensitive avalanche photodiode.

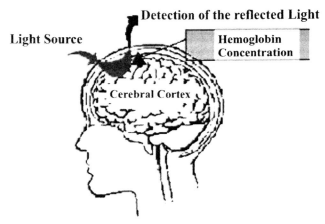

Figure 1. Near-infrared light injected from the scalp passes through the cerebral cortex and is detected at the scalp level.

The brain activity is characterized by the firing of neurons, which results in active energy metabolism and this causes increase in blood volume to supply glucose and oxygen to the tissues. Therefore, the change in concentration of hemoglobin is used as an index to determine the brain activity. The hemoglobin levels are displayed in *mmol·mm* unit of volume. This unit of measurement is described by the following formula:

$$(mmol \cdot mm) = Hb_{mw} * O_{PL} \qquad (1)$$

Where HB_{mw} is the molecular weight in mol and O_{PL} represents the optical path length in mm.

The unit of *mmol*mm* expressed here is a product of the change in concentration of hemoglobin and the optical path length. Based on the absorption property of hemoglobin for near-infrared light used in this equipment, changes in concentration of oxy- and deoxy-hemoglobin are calculated from the changes in the received signals. Consequently, they correspond to the change in concentration of hemoglobin in a living body [Hitachi manual, 2002].

The reflected light is measured every 0.1 seconds, and the current measured data is subtracted from the former to obtain the concentration change of hemoglobin. The intensity of the reflected light depends on the concentration of two kinds of hemoglobin (oxy and dexoy). Two kinds of laser diodes (780nm and 830nm) are used in order to separate the two kinds of hemoglobin concentration. It is necessary for the spectral line width of each diode to be narrow enough to determine precisely the two results. That is reason behind using laser diodes. How active specific regions of the brain are determined by the OTS by continuously monitoring the blood hemoglobin levels, while having the examinee do some specific action or task. [Hitachi website, 2004].

2.2 System Configuration

The OTS consists of three parts as illustrated in Figure 2. The first is the light source, which generates laser beams of 780nm and 830nm through optical fibers. The second is the probe, which directs the modulated laser light onto the examinee's head and receives the reflection back from the head. Reflected light is then sent to the avalanche photodiodes through the fibers. The third is the controller, which converts the optical signals into the electrical ones, analyses the data and then displays the results.

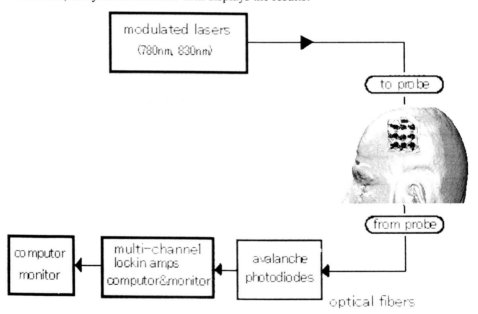

Figure 2. System configuration for OTS

The probe consists of a soft plastic board on which the optical fibers are mounted. Two 3x3 probe sets as illustrated in Figure 3 are used to measure two brain hemispheres simultaneously. Each probe set contains 9 electrodes and can record up to 12 channels of measurement simultaneously.

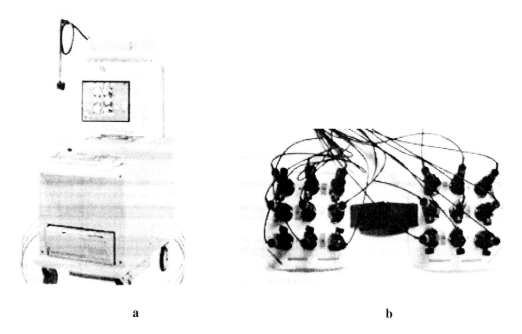

a   b

Figure 3. a) OTS equipment used b) 3x3 Probe

2. MAGNETIC RESONANCE IMAGING (MRI)

MRI provides high quality anatomical images of the human body without invasive radiation or infusion of radioactive substances. It uses the principles of Nuclear Magnetic Resonance (NMR) phenomenon. NMR occurs when the nuclei of certain atoms are immersed in a static magnetic field and exposed to a second oscillating magnetic field.

MRI is based upon the interaction between an applied magnetic field and nuclei of hydrogen atoms present in the human body. The hydrogen atom is an ideal atom for MRI because its nucleus has a single proton. Each proton behaves as a small magnet with a magnetic moment that has a magnitude and direction. The magnetic moments of the individual hydrogen nuclei present in the human body are oriented in random directions. When a strong magnetic field is applied to the human body, the nuclei align their magnetic moments in the direction of the magnetic field as shown in Figure 4 [Hendee and Ritenour, 2002].

Another effect of the applied magnetic field is that it produces additional spin of the magnetic moments so that protons precess with the axis of rotation. Precession is a second order motion; it is the rotation of a rotating object. The frequency f of precession of a proton in units of megahertz (10^6 cycles or rotations per second) depends upon its gyromagnetic ratio γ (in megahertz per tesla) which is constant for each nucleus and the strength of the magnetic field B (in tesla, T). This relationship is described by Larmor equation

$$f = \gamma \, \mathbf{B} \tag{2}$$

Main Magnetic Field

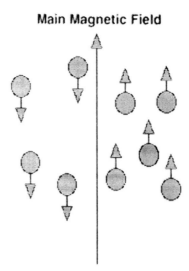

Figure 4: Hydrogen atoms aligned with the magnetic field

When hydrogen nuclei are exposed to a second time varying magnetic field of an electromagnetic wave that has a frequency that matches the precession of protons in a particular magnetic field, it is said to be in resonance. This is the origin of the term magnetic resonance. Protons that precess so that their magnetic fields intersect the plane of a nearby coil will induce an electric current in the coil. This current is the MR signal induced in the receiver coil. When the radio frequency wave is switched off, the signal decays away. This decay is the result of the return of protons to the state that existed before the radio wave was applied. This is known as relaxation of protons. There are two basic relaxation processes. One process involves a return of the protons to their original alignment with the magnetic field. This process is called longitudinal or spin- lattice relaxation and is characterized by time constant T1. The other process is called transverse or spin-spin relaxation and is characterized by time constant T2 [Rabi et al, 1939; Bloembergen, 1948].

Thus, the clinical MRI is obtained by placing the subject to be imaged in a large magnet and the short-wave radio frequency pulses are applied to generate the MR signal that can be quantified and captured by the computer.

3. DATA ACQUISITION

Eight healthy subjects between 20-25 years of old were selected to do an anatomical MRI exam and a finger tapping test using the ETG 100 OTS, under expert clinical supervision. The finger tapping test is a general demonstration of the cerebrum functional measurement, which is not affected by a surrounding environment, and is one of the most consistent tests administered. Measuring a motor function with the OTS consisted of the following steps:

- A repetitive measurement of stimulus (finger tapping) and rest is done alternately and the variation of the amount of hemoglobin against a state of rest is measured.

- Since the rise time of blood flow increase at motor area is around 5 sec, the stimulus time is set to fifteen seconds, which includes rise time and enough spare time.

- A rest time after the stimulus need to be longer than the sum of the time when the blood flow settles down completely and the time used for the base line compensation. This rest time is set to 45 seconds.

During the stimulus, the subject taps his/her finger (tapping order: forefinger-little finger). Stimulus and resting periods are repeated five times, alternately. In all the subject studies, the probe holder is attached to the motor area as shown in Figure 5, and aligned so that probe number (Blue5) is located at C3 scalp electrode and probe number (Blue1) is located at C4 scalp electrode, in accordance with the electrode placement of the standard 10-20 system. The above settings were used for all the subjects.

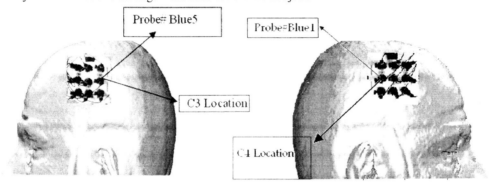

Figure 5: Holder attached to the motor area

Integral analysis is performed on all subjects, during which all the stimulation periods of finger tapping are averaged together. This type of analysis will enhance the statistical output of the signal. In case an artifact (such as body movement) occurs during measurement, the stimulation period that corresponds to that artifact is removed from the integral analysis. MR images were acquired using the Philips Intera MRI scanner. High resolution T1 weighted images were obtained.

4. ALGORITHM DEVELOPMENT PROCESS: CONSTRUCTION OF THE TOPOGRAPHIC IMAGE

In order to map the changes in brain activation (hemoglobin concentration), it is necessary to know their accurate locations. The white circles shown in Figure 6 represent the positions of source points (transmitters), and the black circles represent detector points position. The point midway between a source point and a detector point is defined as a measured point or channel denoted here by numbered squares. The measured points detect both the oxy- and deoxy-hemoglobin change and are denoted here by numbered squares, where each position is decided by the electrodes position.

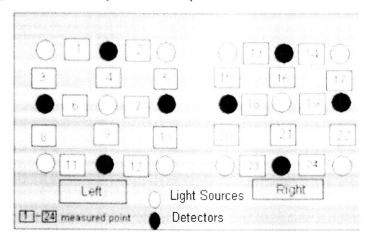

Figure 6. Probes placement architecture

The Topographic image is thus created from the samples of data generated by the OTS. The sampled points or measured points:[ch1, ch2, ch3, ch4, ch5, ch6, ch7, ch8, ch9, ch10, ch11, ch12] are placed in an array for further analysis. In order to construct a square array (4x4), the missing points will be interpolated using averaging interpolation, which consists of averaging between the closest measured points as given by the matrix of measured points (M_{mp}) below:

$$M_{mp} = \begin{cases} \dfrac{ch8 + ch3}{2} & ch3 & ch1 & \dfrac{ch1 + ch2}{2} \\ ch8 & ch6 & ch4 & ch2 \\ ch11 & ch9 & ch7 & ch5 \\ \dfrac{ch11 + ch12}{2} & ch12 & ch10 & \dfrac{ch5 + ch10}{2} \end{cases} \tag{3}$$

Several interpolation methods have been explored, but the best interpolation results were achieved using Spline interpolation. Figure 7 provides few examples for comparative purposes; the black stars are the measured points. The (4x4) M_{mp} matrix is interpolated to form a smooth 32x32 pixel array, and the resulting matrix is displayed as a topographic image as given in Figure 8. The red color (darker gray) reflects the region of activation.

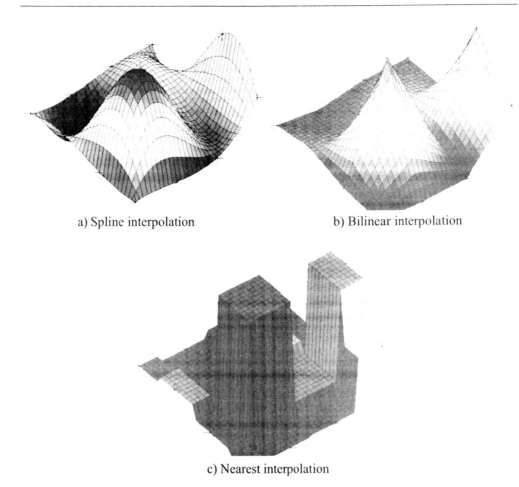

a) Spline interpolation

b) Bilinear interpolation

c) Nearest interpolation

Figure 7. Polynomial fitting of measured points (black stars) using spline, bilinear, and nearest interpolation

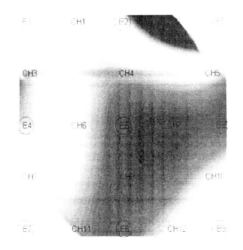

Figure 8. Topographic image displaying the oxyhemoglobin.

6. CONSTRUCTION OF 3D HEAD MODEL FROM ANATOMICAL MRI SLICES

A 3D head model is generated from the structural MRI slices, and in order to further ensure a smooth 3D rendering of the MRI slices, the basic global thresholding algorithm was used. The objective of this latter task is to exclude background from object. This threshold is automatically computed for each subject.

Image segmentation has received considerable attention in literature [Cheriet et al, 1998; Pal et al, 1993; Sahoo et al, 1988; Trier et al, 1995; Trier et al, 1995]. One way to threshold an image is to partition its histogram by using a single global threshold. Segmentation is then accomplished by scanning the image pixel by pixel and labeling each pixel as object or background, depending on whether the gray level of that pixel is greater or less than the obtained threshold value. The success of this method depends on how well the histogram can be partitioned.

The following algorithm has been used to obtain a global threshold T for the entire volume of MRI slices:

- An initial estimate for the threshold (T) is selected to be midway between the maximum and minimum gray levels.
- The image is segmented using the initial threshold T. This will produce two groups of pixels: G1 consisting of all pixels with gray level values > T and G2 consisting of pixels with values $\leq$ T.
- The average gray level values μ_1 and μ_2 are computed for the pixels in regions G1 and G2.
- The new threshold T is then computed as: $T = \frac{1}{2}(\mu_1 + \mu_2)$

Steps 2 through 4 are repeated until the difference in T in successive iterations is smaller than a predefined parameter $\varepsilon_0 \approx 0$ [Gonzalez and Woods, 2002].

This algorithm was used to determine a global threshold for a volume of MRI slices for each subject, where the initial value of T in all the cases (seven patients) is the value midway between the maximum and minimum gray levels. The histogram for the entire volume of MRI for one subject is shown in Figure 9.

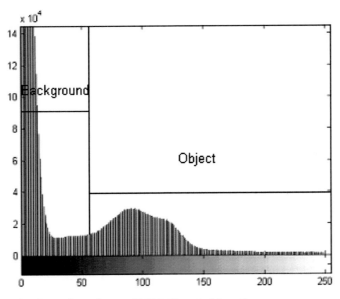

Figure 9. Histogram for the entire volume of MRI slices (subject 1)

The thresholds obtained for all subjects using global thresholding are shown in Table 1. Since thresholding is a rather subjective process, global thresholding provides a suitable way to search for an optimized threshold for each given set of MRI slices of each patient.

Table 1: Global thresholding results for the seven patients

Patients	Basic Global Thresholding
Subject #1	62.23
Subject #2	69.60
Subject #3	74.38
Subject #4	97.71
Subject #5	74.21
Subject #6	68.31
Subject #7	59.00
Subject#8	82.71

Figure 10, shows an example of segmentation based on global thresholding. Figure 10a is the original image (transaxial slice of MRI). Figure10b is the image histogram. Application of the iterative algorithm for this particular case resulted in a threshold value of 97.71. Figure 10c shows the segmented image after thresholding. As expected from the separation of modes in the histogram, the segmentation between object and background was effective.

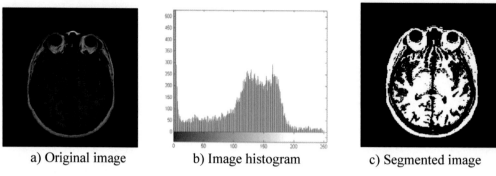

a) Original image   b) Image histogram   c) Segmented image

Figure 10. Displaying a transaxial slice before and after segmentation

Using Matlab software, a volume rendering as shown in Figure 11 is created based on "Marching cubes: 3D surface construction algorithm" [Lorensen and Cline,1987] after using the computed threshold on the MRI slices.

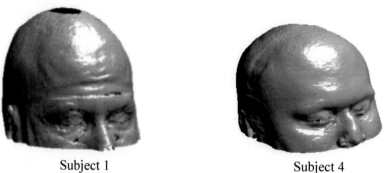

Subject 1   Subject 4

Figure 11: Head models constructed from a volume of anatomical slices.

7. DETECTION OF THE PROBES LOCATION

An algorithm is developed that will first identify the regions on the 3D head model from which the topographic image generated by OTS was taken. The algorithm is structured as follows: the user is asked to identify the location of the left and right ear, nasion and inion by clicking on the head model. Then by using the geometry of the "10-20 system" of electrode placement as portrayed in Figures 12 and Figure 13, an automated algorithm will identify the location of scalp electrodes C3,C4, and Cz on the head model, where C3 is equivalent to probe#Blue5, and C4 is equivalent to probe#Blue1. Then, the remaining probes will be determined by pixel walking on the head model a distance of 2.6 cm (in accordance to 2D projections of the electrode spacing) in perpendicular direction (up and down) from C3 and (up and down) from C4. Electrodes C3 and C4 are used here as startup positions. After determining the location of the probes all the pixels that fall within the boundaries of the probes are determined, extracted and stored in an array. The topographic images are then warped to the extracted pixels.

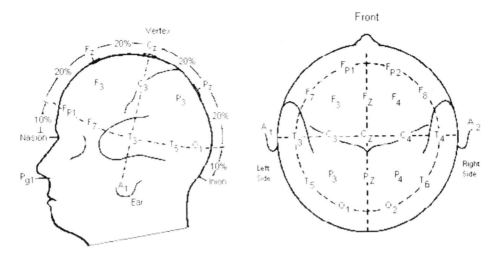

Figure 12. "10-20 system" electrode placement architecture

The computational steps of the algorithm are summarized next. Figure 13 is used as a support illustration for the description provided.

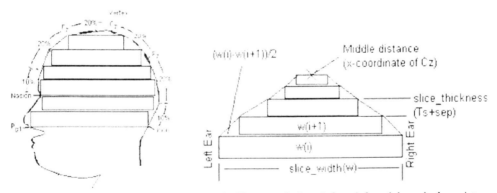

a) Illustrates frontal length (Nasion-inion)   b) illustrates the length from left to right auricular points.

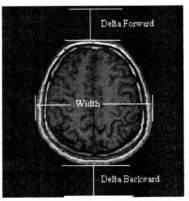

c) A transaxial slice showing delta forward, delta backward, and width of slice

Figure 13. Illustrating the geometry used on the MRI slice.

Step 1: Determining the transaxial position of electrodes C3 and C4

Using Figure 13 as a reference illustration, the following measures are used to determine on which transaxial slice scalp electrodes C3 and C4 are located.

- The width of each transaxial slice is determined and stored as variable w.

- To compute the circumference $C_{LR}(N_s)$ from the left ear to the right ear, the following equaton was developed to compute a partial sum over a number of continuous slices:

$$C_{lR}(i) = \sum_{k=1}^{i} 2 * \sqrt{(T_s + \Delta_s)^2 + \left(\frac{w(k) - w(k+1)}{2}\right)^2} \tag{4}$$

where i indicates which transaxial slice is used, $w(i)$ is the width of slice number i, N_s is the total number of transaxial slices, Δ_s is the separation distance between the transaxial slices and T_s is the slice thickness. For the final slice, just the width of the slice is added to the circumference $C_{LR}(N_s)$. When $i = N_s$, equation (4) returns the circumference from the left to the right ear.

- To determine the 30 % distance, the following equation is used:

$$F(i) = \sum_{k=1}^{i} (C_{LR}(k)/2) \tag{5}$$

In equation (5), i and k represent slice numbers, with $i = 1, 2, ..., N_s$.

- Equation (6) is used to compute F_{rel} as:

$$F_{rel}(i) = \frac{F(i)}{2 * F(N_s)} \tag{6}$$

With both F(i) and F(Ns) computed with the use of Equation (5).

- Check when $F_{rel}(i) = 0.3$, which is 30% of the total circumference C_{LR}. The value of i when this condition is satisfied will correspond to the transaxial slice where the scalp electrodes C3, and C4 are located.

Step 2: Locating the X-coordinate of scalp electrode Cz

The transaxial slice where $F_{rel} = 0.5$ is determined, and this corresponds to the z-coordinate of Cz, which is midway between auricular A1 and A2 points. Then, the center of the slice is located and used as the x-coordinate for the scalp electrode Cz.

Step 3: Locating the Y-coordinate for scalp electrode Cz

The following algorithm will calculate the distance from the nasion to inion, in order to determine the location of the y-coordinate for Cz.

The frontal length (i.e. the length from the nasion to the upper top slice) is computed using equation (7) as follows:

$$frontallen gth[Nasion \rightarrow final\_slice] = \sum_{i=nasion}^{final\_slice} hyplength(i) \qquad (7)$$

where *hyplength* represents the length of the hypotenuse and is computed in this geometry as:

$$hyplength(i) = \sqrt{(\Delta F(i+1) - \Delta F(i))^2 + Ts^2} \qquad (8)$$

ΔF is the distance from the top of each transaxial slice to the edge or the Delta forward in Figure 13.c. The height of the final slice is computed and added to the total length.

Similarly, the occipital length (the length from the final slice to inion) is computed by replacing (ΔF) with (ΔB) in equation (8). The total length is computed by adding the frontal and occipital sums. As a result, the length from the nasion to scalp electrode Cz is equal to half the total length nasion to inion.

This algorithm is repeated until 50% of the total length (nasion-inion) is located. The index of the sum will correspond to the slice number where the scalp electrode Cz is located and the pixel where the length is 50% will now be the y-coordinate.

Step 4: Locating all the pixels that fall within the probe holder

After locating the coordinates of the scalp electrodes C3, C4, and Cz, then the remaining probes will be determined by pixel walking on the head model a distance of 2.6 cm in perpendicular direction from C3 and C4 as shown in Figure 14. After determining the location of the probes, all the pixels that fall within the boundaries of the probe holder are determined, extracted and stored in an array. Then the 2D topographic images are warped to the extracted pixels as illustrated in Figure 15.

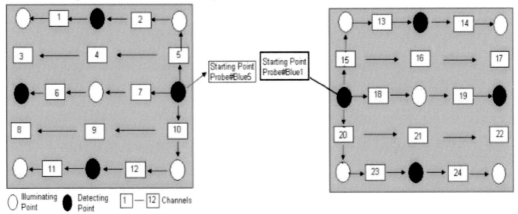

a) Left probe holder   b) Right probe holder

Figure 14. Probe architecture

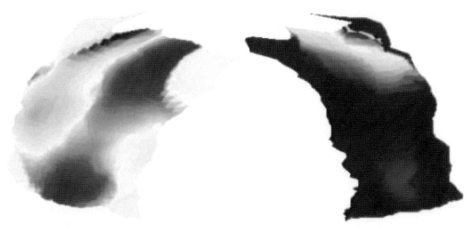

Figure 15. Warped topographic images

The integration of these warped topographic images with head models are examplified in Figure 16 for 3 different subjects.

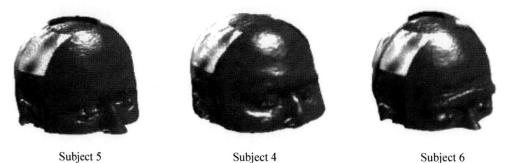

Subject 5   Subject 4   Subject 6
Figure 16. Integration of topographic images with MRI

8. EXTRACTION OF BRAIN IMAGES

Automated software BET (Brain Extraction Tool) for segmenting the MRI head images into brain and non-brain has been used successfully before [Smith, 2002]. BET software "uses a deformable model which evolves to fit the brain's surface by the application of a set of locally adaptive model forces". Segmenting the brain from non-brain tissue allows for the fusion of topographic images with the brain. The FSL software interface is as displayed in Figure 17.

The BET tool box is used to extract brain from the MRI data. After extracting the brain, 3D reconstruction is performed. The results obtained are depicted in Figure 18.

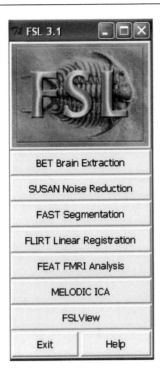

Figure 17. FSL software interface

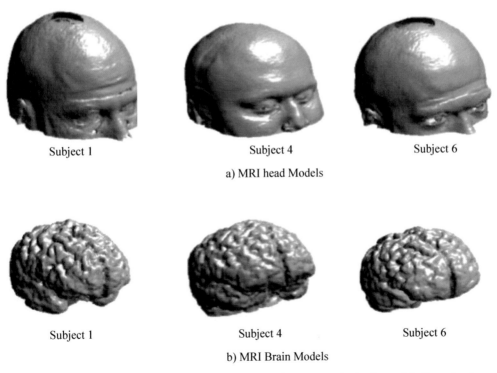

a) MRI head Models

b) MRI Brain Models

Figure 18. Examples where the BET software was used to extract the brain models from the few of the subjects used in this study.

9. INTEGRATING TOPOGRAPHIC MAPS WITH BRAIN MODEL

After extracting the brain from MRI data, the topographic maps that were registered to the head model, are then projected to the brain model. An illustration of this projection is given in Figure 19.

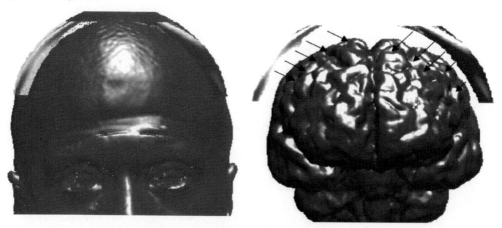

Figure 19. Integrating topographic maps with the head model and brain model before projection

Firstly, the scalp electrodes C3 and C4 located on the skull of the head are projected to the brain according to the algorithm provided below, using illustration of Figure 20 as a reference:

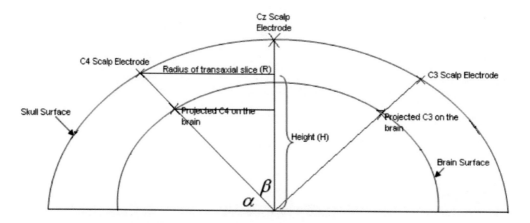

Figure 20. Projecting the scalp electrodes (C3, C4) to the brain model

- The relative ratio R_{rel} is computed, which is the ratio of the height over the radius of the transaxial slice where the scalp electrodes C3-C4 are located as in Figure 21.

$$R_{rel} = \frac{Height}{Radius} \qquad (9)$$

- For each transaxial brain slice $bs(i)$ starting from the top, compute the radius of bs(i) (*radius_bs(i)*) height for each transaxial slice (*height_bs(i)*)

- If $\dfrac{height\_bs(i)}{radius\_bs(i)} = R_{rel}$ then the ith transaxial slice hits the projection line and the projected scalp electrodes C3 and C4 will be located at this transaxial slice, if not increment i and test again.

After projecting the scalp electrodes C3 and C4 to the brain model, the rest of the pixels are determined following the same algorithm that was used at the scalp level. Then the topographic images are warped to the extracted pixels. The integration of the warped topographic images with the brain model is illustrated in Figure 21.

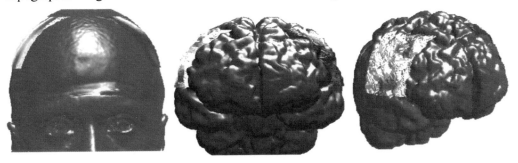

Figure 21. Integrating topographic maps with head and brain models after projection

10. VALIDATION OF THE RESULTS

In order to verify the results obtained, a comparison is made between the fiducial markers (Vitamin E) placed on the patients head during the MRI test to localize the probes location and an automated computer program that will detect the probes position. The numbers on the head model as given in Figure 22 represent the location of the probes as determined by the computer program, while the round circles represent the fiducial markers. The integration of topographic maps to anatomical MRI is illustrated in Figure 23.

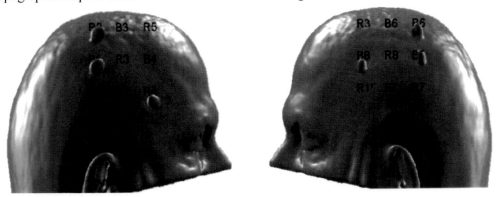

Figure 22. Head model with fiducial markers to verify the location of the electrode

The Euclidean distance is used as a measure of error between the fiducial markers (x_f, y_f, z_f) and the computed electrodes position (x_c, y_c, z_c) as illustrated in table 2.

Table 2: Calculating the Error between fiducial markers and the computed location of Electrodes

Electrode#	Computed Position of Electrodes (x_c, y_c, z_c)	Fiducial Marker (x_f, y_f, z_f)	Euclidean Distance (mm)
R6	(165,152,70)	(168,152,69)	3.428
B5	(206,152,57)	(204,152,58)	2.71
R10	(203,96,44)	(205,96,49)	9.97
R2	(91, 152,70)	(84,144,69)	10.15
B1	(60,152,57)	(56,149,55)	6

The integration of topographic maps and anatomical MRI at the scalp and cortical level is illustrated in Figure 23. A graphical user interface was developed [Mourad et al, 2005] that integrates the proposed modalities with the capability of mapping the functional areas of the brain by displaying a video of topographic maps on the MRI head model.

11. CONCLUSION

This study introduced a new integrated approach between two different modalities, namely MRI and OTS. The objective was to develop an automated algorithm that will locate on the 3D brain model the activation that is seen by the OTS, which allow us to display of a movie of topographic maps on the head model. The algorithm involved the integration of key imaging techniques coupled with 3D rendering and a new integration process that allowed for the OTS image to be superimposed correctly on volumetric MRI slices.

This innovative approach as structured established a framework that has consolidated and validated results from two different sensing modalities by introducing a unique localization approach that has taken results at the scalp levels and projected them into the cortical surface. Results have shown that such integration is most effective, yielding accurate localization results for all the seven subjects involved in this study.

The validation process proved very useful by making use of fiducial markers (Vitamin E) placed on the patients head during the MRI data acquisition. Through such markers it was possible to effectively verify the results obtained through the automated algorithm with the actual probes positions. The Euclidean distance that was used as a measure of error between the fiducial markers and the computed electrodes position showed relatively low errors.

Foreseeable applications of this method will come in support of other diagnostic studies performed in our earlier work [Mirkovic and Adjouadi, 2003; Adjouadi et al, 2004; Cabrerizo et al, 2005], and will serve researchers and clinicians as an integrated multi-modal sensory-based research and diagnostic platform.

Subject 1:

Subject 2:

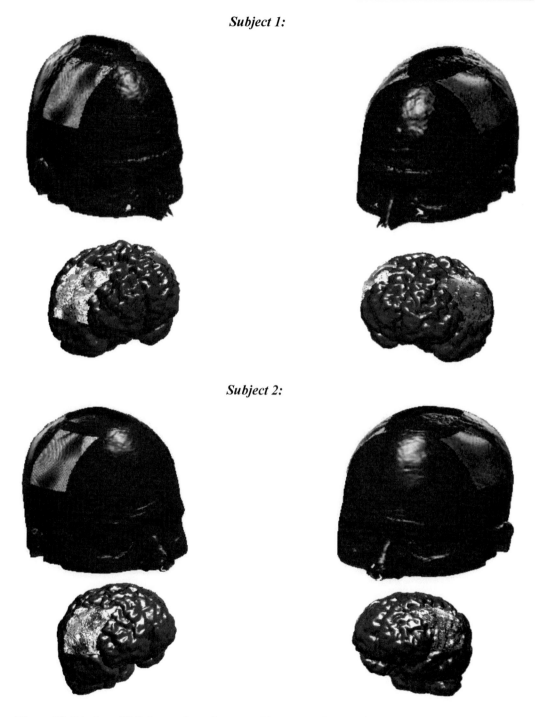

Figure 23. Display of 3-D integration of topographic maps and anatomical MRI

Subject 3:

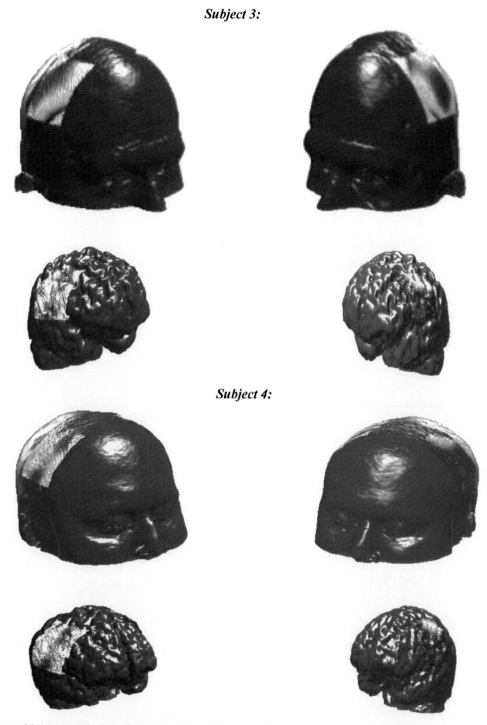

Subject 4:

Figure 23 (cont.). Display of 3D integration of topographic maps and anatomical MRI

Subject 5:

Subject 6:

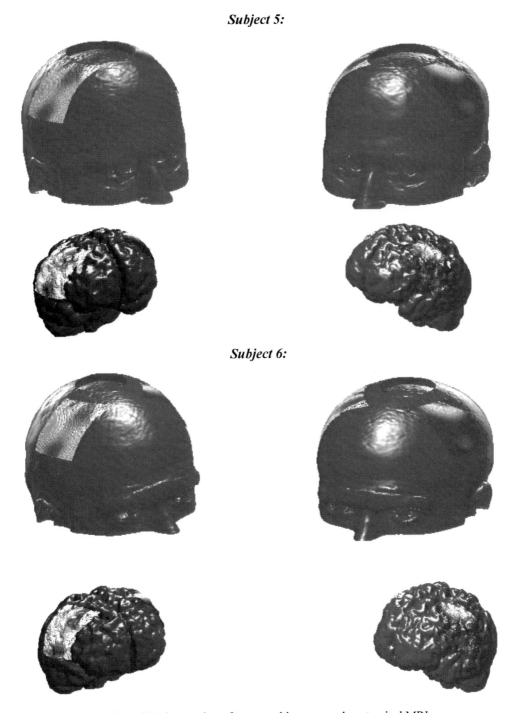

Figure 23 (cont.). Display of 3D integration of topographic maps and anatomical MRI

ACKNOWLEDGMENTS

This research was supported by the National Science Foundation Grants EIA-9906600, HRD- 0317692, CNS 042615, and the Office of Naval Research Grant N00014-99-1-0952. The support of Miami Children's Hospital is greatly appreciated.

REFERENCES

Adjouadi, M., Cabrerizo, M., Yaylali, I., and Jayakar, P., "Interpreting EEG Functional Brain Activity", *IEEE Potentials*, pp. 8-13, Feb/March Issue 2004.

Arridge, S.R., "Optical tomography in medical imaging", *Inverse Problems* 15, R1-R53 (1999).

Bloembergen, N., Purcell, E., and Pound, R., "Relaxation effects in nuclear magnetic resonance absorption", *Physiol. Rev*, 73:679-712

Boas, D. A., Dale, A. M. and. Franceschini, M. A, "Diffuse optical imaging of brain activation: approaches to optimizing image sensitivity, resolution, and accuracy", *Neuroimage* 23, S275-288 (2004).

Boas, D. A. and Dale, A. M., "Simulation study of magnetic resonance imaging-guided cortically constrained diffuse optical tomography of human brain function", *Appl. Opt.* 44, 1957-68 (2005).

Cabrerizo, M., Adjouadi, M., Ayala, M., Nunez, K., Jayakar, P., and Yaylali, I., "Integrated Analysis of EEG Functional Brain Mapping Based on an Auditory-Comprehension Process Augmented Through Topographical Maps and a New Eigensystem Study", *Brain Topography*, Vol. 17 (3), pp. 151-163, 2005.

Cheriet, M., Said, J., and Suen, C.Y, "A Recursive Thresholding Technique for Image Segmentation", *IEEE Trans. Image Processing,* Vol 7, no 6, pp 918-921, 1998.

Frostig, RD., Lieke, EE, Ts'o, DY, Grinwald, A., "Cortical functional architecture and local coupling between neuronal activity and microcirculation revealed by vivo high-resolution optical imaging of intrinsic signals", *Proc Natl Acad Sci USA* 87:6082-6086, 1990.

Gonzalez, R., Woods, R., *Digital Image Processing*, Prentice Hall, New Jersey; 2nd edition, 2002.

Hendee, W. R. E., Ritenour , R. R., *Medical Imaging Physics*, Wiley-Liss, New York, Fourth edition, 2002.

Hitachi Medical System America, INC (2004, August 15). [Online]. Available: *http://www.hitachimed.com/products/optical_configuration.asp.*

Kennan, R., Kim, D., Maki, A., Koizumi, H. and Constable R., "Non-Invasive Assessment of Language Lateralization by Transcranial Near Infrared Optical Topography and Functional MRI", *Human Brain Mapping*, 16:183-189, 2002.

Kennan, R., Horovitz , S., Maki, A., Yamashita, Y., Koizumi, K., and Gore, J., "Simultaneous recording of event-related auditory oddball response using transcranial near infrared optical topography and surface EEG", *Neuro Image* 16, 587-592, 2002.

Kleinschmidt, A., Obrig, H., Requardt, M., Merboldt, K. D., Dirnagl, U., Villringer, A., and Frahm, J.,"Simultaneous recording of cerebral blood oxygenation changes during human brain activation by magnetic resonance imaging and near-infrared spectroscopy," *J. Cereb. Blood Flow Metab.* 16, 817–826 (1996).

Lorensen, W., and Cline, H., "Marching cubes: A high resolution 3D surface construction algorithm," *Computer Graphics* 21(4), pp. 163--169, 1987.

Mayhew, J., Zhao, L., Hou, Y., Berwick, J., Askew, S., Zheng, Y., Coffey, P., "Spectroscopic investigation of reflectance changes in the barrel cortex following whisker stimulation", *Adv Exp Med Biol* 454:139-148, 1998.

Mirkovic, N., Adjouadi, M., Yaylali, I., and Jayakar P., "3-D Source Localization of Epileptic Interictal Spikes", *Brain Topography Journal*, Vol. 16, No.2, pp. 111-119, Jan. 2003.

Mourad, M., Adjouadi, M., Yaylali, Y., "A projection Approach of Optical Topographic Maps to the Cortical Surface of the Brain", Proceedings of the 2nd International IEEE EMBS Conference on Neural Engineering, pp. 13-16, Arlington, Virginia, U.S.A, March 16-19, 2005.

Mourad, M., Adjouadi, M., Yaylali, I., Ayala, M. and Rishe, N. "An Interface for Analyzing and Integrating Different Imaging Modalities", *WSEAS Transactions on Signal Processing*, Issue 3, Vol. 1, pp. 392-397, December 2005.

Hitachi Medical Corporation , *Optical Topography System Operation Manual*, 2002.

Pal, N., and Pal, S., "A review on image segmentation techniques", *Pattern Recognit.*, vol 26, pp. 1277-1294, 1993.

Rabi, I.I., Millman, S., Kush, P., and Zacharias, J., "Molecular beam resonance method for measuring nuclear magnetic moments", *Physiol. Rev*, 55:526-535, 1939

Sahoo, P., Soltani, S., and Wong, A., "SURVEY: A survey of thresholding techniques", *Comput. Vis. Graph. Image Process.*, vol. 41, pp. 233–260, 1988.

Smith, A., "BET: Brain Extraction Tool", FMRIB technical Report TR00SMS2b, 2002 [online]. Available at: *http://www.fmrib.ox.ac.uk/analysis/research/bet/bet/*

Strangman, G., Culver, J.P., Thompson, J.H., and Boas, D.A., "A quantitative comparison of simultaneous BOLD fMRI and NIRS recording during functional brain activation," *Neuroimage*, **17**, 719-731 (2002).

Trier, O. D., and Jain, A. K., "Goal-directed evaluation of binarization methods", *IEEE Trans. Pattern Anal. Machine Intell.*, vol. 17, pp.1191–1201, Dec. 1995.

Trier, O. D and Taxt, T., "Evaluation of binarization methods for document images," *IEEE Trans. Pattern Anal. Machine Intell.*, vol. 17, pp. 312–315, Mar. 1995.

Zhang, X. , Toronov, V.Y., and Webb, A.G. "Simultaneous integrated diffuse optical tomography and functional magnetic resonance imaging of the human brain", Opt. Express 13, 5513-5521 (2005), *http://www.opticsexpress.org/abstract.cfm?URI=OPEX-13-14-5513*

INDEX

Q

R

S

W

X

Y